Contents

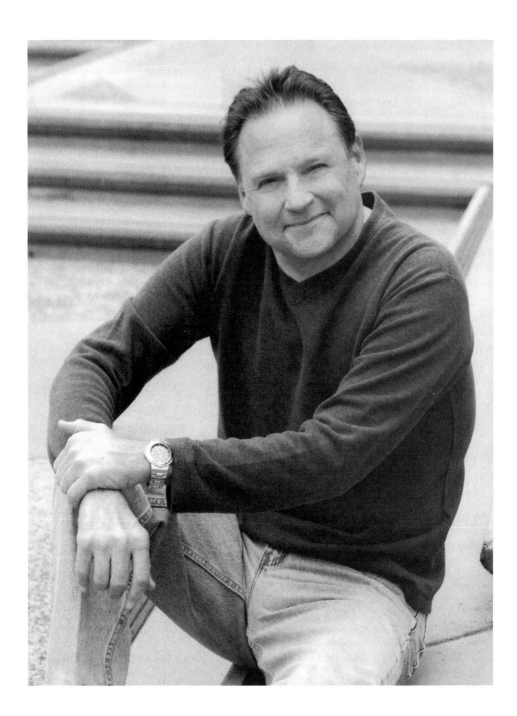

Confessions of a Couch Potato

(Or, If I'm So **Skinny,** Why Do I Still Feel Like **Flounder?**)

Stephen Furst

American Diabetes Association.

Cure • Care • Commitment℠

Director, Book Publishing, John Fedor; *Book Acquisitions,* Sherrye Landrum; *Editor,* Sherrye Landrum; *Production Manager,* Peggy M. Rote; *Cover Design,* Rikki Campbell; *Printer,* Transcontinental Printing

Printed in Canada
1 3 5 7 9 10 8 6 4 2

The suggestions and information contained in this publication are generally consistent with the *Clinical Practice Recommendations* and other policies of the American Diabetes Association, but they do not represent the policy or position of the Association or any of its boards or committees. Reasonable steps have been taken to ensure the accuracy of the information presented. However, the American Diabetes Association cannot ensure the safety or efficacy of any product or service described in this publication. Individuals are advised to consult a physician or other appropriate health care professional before undertaking any diet or exercise program or taking any medication referred to in this publication. Professionals must use and apply their own professional judgment, experience, and training and should not rely solely on the information contained in this publication before prescribing any diet, exercise, or medication. The American Diabetes Association—its officers, directors, employees, volunteers, and members—assumes no responsibility or liability for personal or other injury, loss, or damage that may result from the suggestions or information in this publication.

∞ The paper in this publication meets the requirements of the ANSI Standard Z39.48-1992 (permanence of paper).

ADA titles may be purchased for business or promotional use or for special sales. To purchase this book in large quantities, or for custom editions of this book with your logo, contact Lee Romano Sequeira, Special Sales & Promotions, at the address below, or at LRomano@diabetes.org or 703-299-2046.

American Diabetes Association
1701 North Beauregard Street
Alexandria, Virginia 22311

Library of Congress Cataloging-in-Publication Data

Furst, Stephen, 1955-
    Confesssions of a couch potato, or, If I'm so skinny, why do I still feel like flounder? / Stephen Furst
        p. cm.
    ISBN 1-58040-144-9 (pbk. : alk. paper)
    1. Non-insulin-dependent diabetes--Diet therapy. I. Title: If I'm so skinny, why do I still feel like flounder?. II. Title.

RC662.18.F87 2002
616.4'620654--dc21   2002026104

Dedication

This book is dedicated to my college acting teacher who told me that the chances of a fat guy making it in Hollywood were pretty slim. "No pun intended," he added. He died of cigarette smoking about 6 years after I starred in my first movie. Also to the commercial agent who turned me down and said, "I'm sorry, they just don't use fat people in commercials." This is the same guy who tried to sell me a washer and dryer years later at Sears, when his agency went under. He offered me free delivery if I made the purchase right then, but I turned him down this time and bought it at a store I had done a commercial for earlier.

To my two sons who made fun of all the crazy recipe concoctions that I created but were always there cheering me on. And to anyone who has ever heard the words "You have such a pretty face, if you could only lose a little weight." This book is for you!

Introduction

This book is not another diet book with calorie counting and measuring. It is the story of a metamorphosis. The transformation of a 320-pound teenager—who considered the "breakfast of champions" to be 6 Big Macs and a diet coke—to a normal-weight, middle-aged man who cooks with anything that is non- or low fat. I don't even

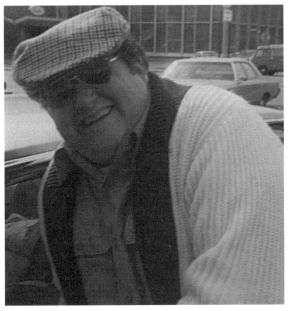

Back in my Big Mac hey-day.

think about it anymore. It just comes naturally. I still enjoy all the foods I used to—minus the fat and sugar. Sugar is usually a no-no for me because I have diabetes... (No, wait, they're telling me that I CAN have sugar, but I have to count the carb in it.) Anyway, I still stuff myself like a pig. Really. I much prefer to eat at buffet restaurants to ensure that I get enough to eat. I'll tell you how you can too and include my recipes for wonderful low-fat and sugar-free goodies. I'll tell you stories of my life of "living large" with the movies for a backdrop. Some will make you laugh till you cry and others will just make you cry, like I did.

I've been making fat jokes about myself ever since I can remember. I've always been overweight, and I wanted to beat everyone else to the punch. The jokes didn't hurt as much if they came from me. I think only professionals should give advice about their area of expertise. Well, take it from me, I am a professional fat person—and dieter. I have probably lost 1,500 pounds in my life. I was an expert at saying how stuffed I am after eating over at someone's house and then making a beeline for the nearest mini-market as soon as I left. I was a pro at making excuses for leaving my shirt on at the beach, or conveniently feeling ill when we played basketball and one team would be the "shirts" and one would be the "skins." I even told the teacher once that it was against my religion to be something called a "skin." When he looked at me with a dumbfounded expression, I just explained that it had something to do with keeping kosher. This book is written for anyone who has struggled with being overweight—which happens to be half the population of the United States.

I once tipped the scales at 320 pounds. Now I weigh 175 pounds and a lot of people have asked me what's my secret. Did I go on the grapefruit diet? Was it Pritikin? Did I sweat to the oldies with Little Richard (oh, I mean Richard Simmons, I always get those guys confused)? Well, to tell you the truth, I am an addict. Yes, that's right. My name is Stephen Furst, and I am an addict! Now all together, "Hello Stephen." I'm a food addict, to be precise. My bourbon is bon bons, my martini is manicotti (with extra cheese). Forget cocaine; bring on the cocoa puffs. Actually, as a child I used to eat Sugar Frosted Flakes with chocolate milk, but I digest, I mean digress.

I sat, I ate, I grew. I felt different from everyone else—like an alien. The looks I received when I was 320 pounds were ones usually reserved for three-eyed monsters, half-man half-woman reptiles, creatures with hideous rolls of skin that sweated profusely and giggled when they walked… Oh, my God, that last one really was me. But for all the years I was treated like an alien, it still didn't motivate me to lose weight.

It is like being an addict of drugs or alcohol—you have to hit bottom and become so disgusted with yourself that there is only one choice left, and I'm not talking about choosing between rocky road or chocolate chip cookie dough. It's the choice between life and death. I didn't want to choose death—besides, I hadn't fully gotten even with my kids for all the stress they caused me through the years. I chose to live! I chose to pick myself up (which really wasn't easy) by the bootstraps and enjoy life as a thin person.

I have accomplished that. The physical part is done. I am thin. All I have left is the mental mountain to climb. Sometimes that can be like trying to conquer Mt. Everest. The title of this book says it all for me. Even though I have gone from a size 52 pants to a meager 34, I still feel like that fat person is just waiting for an ideal opportunity to come out and scream, "Surprise! It's me. Let's go get a banana split to celebrate my freedom." Yes indeed, that alien is inside me waiting to get out. When I sat in the make-up chair on the set of *Babylon 5*, and my make-up artist transformed me into an alien, a certain sadness came over me. I lived 40 years as an alien from the planet Lard. I tried to escape more times than you can imagine. Every time I would start to head for my independence, I was called back by my weakness. I finally broke free.

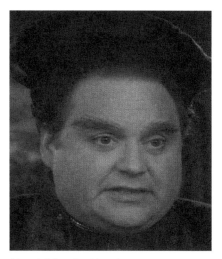

Not Jabba the Hut, but a reasonable facsimile! (*Babylon 5*)

There were a lot of funny and, sometimes, sad events that took place growing up and living all my life as an obese person. The measures I would take to make sure I had enough food to satisfy my cravings may amaze you, or it may sound familiar.

I want to share with you the recipes I came up with to accomplish my goal of growing thin. I made up substitutions for everything, from a complete Thanksgiving dinner with all the trimmings to barbecue sauce and desserts like cheesecake. I never felt deprived because I continued to eat the things that I truly loved, and still love today. I just made up low-fat or no-fat substitutions and ate till I was full. For me, that's what made sense. Eat, feel full, lose weight.

Everyone is so deadly serious about weight—there aren't many funny diet books out there. So, I'm going to share my thoughts, laughs, embarrassing situations, and the tears in my life as the alien that I am. Now, curl up with a bowl of my butter-topped movie theater popcorn (page 90) and enjoy the rest of the book.

Chapter One

Working My Way to the Bottom

To me, saying that you've hit bottom means you can't go any lower. Sheer inertia prevents you from sinking any lower. But the one thing about personal bottoms is that they are always adjustable—until you've reached the point of the ultimate bottom; the bottom that you have no control over, which, of course, is death.

When I was 17, my father died from complications of diabetes. He was 47. I found out the same year that I had type 2 diabetes as well. You'd think that would have been enough for me to finally wake up and smell the bear claws. And to top it all off, I had one of the most embarrassing moments of my obese life to help push me one step closer to the bottom.

It was the summertime. I lived in Norfolk, Virginia. There was a girl in my high school (I'll call her Bonnie to protect the innocent) that I had a fancy for. She was not very popular and definitely not what you would call "the homecoming queen" type. For those reasons, I thought there might be a slight chance she wouldn't laugh in my face if I asked her out. This was in July. By the end of August, I still had not asked her out. Rejection was something for which I had a low threshold. One day I decided this was going to be the day of no return. There was only one more weekend left in the summer. School was starting, and then it would be too late, or so I convinced myself. I picked up the phone and dialed her number. It rang. So I did what any other 300-pound coward would do—I hung up. I socked myself in the head a couple of times and pressed redial on the phone. It rang. Once, twice, and then, "Hello." The voice of Bonnie's mother sounded in my ear.

From the depths of my soul, I mustered up enough nerve to say, "Is Bonnie there?"

"Hold on, I'll get her," she replied. I heard the phone go down on the tile kitchen counter. What probably was only fifteen seconds or so, seemed liked fifteen years as Bonnie made her way to the phone. I had all these thoughts running through my head. I saw my life flash before my eyes several times. I imagined her laughing hysterically as I asked her out. I imagined us at the altar getting married and living "happily ever after," complete with two fat, ugly kids. By now I could hear her footsteps coming closer to the phone. This was it! There was no turning back. Now her footsteps sounded as loud as an elephant stampeding through the brush. She picked up the phone and then it fell out of her hand smashing against the tile. I was deafened by the sound. Then I heard her scramble for the phone. This gave me another five second reprieve from being laughed at and hearing the resounding, "YOU'VE GOT TO BE KIDDING, TUBBY."

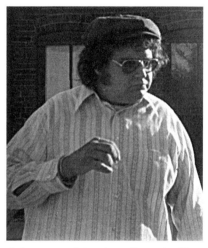

A few years later, in college, I still remember with embarrassment.

"Hello." Bonnie sounded like a princess. The fact that I couldn't actually see her helped the fantasy quite a bit.

"Hi Bonnie, this is Stephen Feuerstein (my real name)." The silence on the other end was as deafening as the earlier phone drop. I knew I had to give her more information than just my name to spark her interest. "I'm the heavyset guy that sat behind you in Mr. McPhee's class last year."

"Oh, yes. Hi." I could tell in her voice that she was thinking, "What the hell does he want with me?" Fear took over my body, all 300 pounds. Once again, I reached within myself to find my inner strength and asked the question. Well, not the question exactly. Unfortunately, I didn't have enough nerve to ask her about the date. Instead, I came out with something stupid. "I was just wondering, if someone asked you to name the capitals of all 50 states, do you think you'd be able to?"

Again, that deafening silence. She finally came up with a definitive answer. "I…uh…really don't know."

"Okay, I was just wondering. I guess I'll talk to you later, goodbye." I hung up the phone before she could even respond to the "goodbye."

I couldn't believe what I had just done. I was so embarrassed and I had to do something to make the embarrassment go away. I needed to seek comfort and solace. I needed a piece of coconut cream pie ASAP. I was not about to let this one little setback impair my life. This was nothing that a couple of double cheeseburgers and fries couldn't handle.

After my misery feast and a few words of encouragement from my best friend, Kenny, I decided to try it again. I dialed up Bonnie that same evening. This time Bonnie answered the phone herself. It didn't even give me the opportunity to have second thoughts.

"Hello?" the princess said.

"Hi, Bonnie, this is Stephen Feuerstein. I'm the heavyset guy that…"

"I know who you are, "she interrupted. "I really haven't had time to work on those capitals you asked about earlier."

I assured her that it wasn't that important, and I could just look them up myself. After a few more moments of talk about the weather and the latest episodes of Bewitched, I finally did it. I said, "Would you like to go out this weekend?...Bonnie, you there?" Again with the deafening silence. But on the other hand, there was no laughter either. I took this as a positive sign. I was just about to hang up the phone and beg my mother to transfer me to another school for my senior year when I heard her voice utter the words that sounded like poetry to my ears.

"Sure. Yeah."

Having been successful so far, I decided not to push my luck any further and immediately hung up the phone. The weekend was quickly approaching. I knew I would have to call her to tell her when I would pick her up and ask her where she would like to go. I didn't want to go to the movies because I didn't want to put any undo pressure on myself—should I hold her hand, should I put my arm around her, should I buy Milk Duds or Good 'N Plenty?

I called her up on Thursday and asked her if she liked amusement parks. With the same poetic flow as before, she replied, "Sure, yeah." It was all set. Saturday night at Ocean View amusement park. I told my mother about my date, and she started crying. I gave her a big hug and told her not to worry, that no woman in the world could ever replace her. She said, "I'm not crying about being replaced. I'm crying because I'm so happy. I thought you would never get a date." With that, she was off to the local bookstore to buy baby naming books for the grandchildren Bonnie and I would undoubtedly give her.

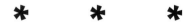

Ocean View amusement park was a small town amusement park. Not anything like the Six Flags parks or Disneyland. These were rides you were sure would go careening off their tracks at any moment. Meanwhile, the ride attendants looked like they just got early parole from Attica.

Bonnie and I strolled down the midway. I knew that I could probably win her heart if I could win the giant panda hanging at the ring toss booth. I slapped down my fifty cents for my three rings and started to become her hero. Five and a half dollars later, I walked away with nothing but a pulled shoulder muscle from all that tossing.

We walked down the midway a little further, turned the corner, and my heart sank. There in front of us was the hawker for the "Guess Your Weight" booth. He was one of those guys that would annoy and ridicule you till you tried to spite him back by winning one of his cheap toys. It didn't matter that the toy was worth about a quarter and it cost a buck to play. He wore one of those microphones around his neck so anyone within 100 yards could hear each and every insult that spewed from his tobacco-stained mouth.

I started to sweat, which, believe it or not, actually came rather easily to me at 300 pounds. What could I do to avoid being totally humiliated to death by a guy who still had handcuff scars on his wrists? The nearest thing to us was a thrill ride called "The Twister." I thought fast on my feet and told Bonnie that I was dying to ride that particular ride. I asked her if she was ready for the thrill of her life. She told me that she didn't kiss on the first date. I assured her that I was just talking about the ride. Just then I heard the hawker show no mercy to a one-legged midget as he hobbled by.

I immediately told Bonnie that it would mean a great deal to me if we could be scared together on The Twister. She, being a shy woman of few words mumbled, "Sure, yeah." I slapped down the money for what was promised as the thrill of my life. It was a very crowded ride. We waited in line for about thirty minutes for our turn to be tossed about by this piece of machinery. Suddenly, I was beginning to question what was a worse fate—being humiliated by the guess-your-weight guy, or trying to carry on a thirty-minute conversation while waiting in line. Finally, it was our turn and all I could think of was how good I was at handling pressure situations. I was able to ask this girl out. I was able to avoid the guess-your-weight guy, and I was able to make enough conversation to fill thirty minutes of wait time for the ride. I was home free. All I had to do was ride the minute and a half ride and call it an evening.

The gate opened for the new riders to board. Bonnie and I went for the green colored car. We lowered ourselves into this sleek futuristic looking car. Over the loud speaker a recorded voice was giving instructions on how to hook up the safety harness in the cars. We pulled the straps over our heads and then the nightmare began. She quickly snapped her belt and was ready to ride. I, on the other hand, quickly learned I was too fat to buckle up. I squirmed in my seat and made several more attempts at safety. I sucked my stomach in until I thought I burst inside, and I was still about three inches short. Three measly inches from a completely successful experience...and then, disaster.

By now, everyone was hooked up and ready. The attendant was making his rounds seeing that everyone was properly strapped in. He got to us and gave a quick tug on Bonnie's belt and then reached over to do mine. I looked up at him, and all I could say was, "I think mine's broken or something." He said, in his most tactful manner, "It ain't broken, you too fat to ride, Mister." I'm sure glad he added that mister at the end or I really would have gotten mad. He then added, "You gonna have to get off and let someone else ride." I slowly slid out of my seat and got out of the car. Bonnie started to unhook, but I insisted that she experience "the thrill of her life." I told her I would wait for her by the exit. I stood by the exit and watched as they led this much thinner guy to occupy the seat that I had to vacate. They rode the ride. It must have been scary because she hung onto the stranger the whole time.

I came home in the biggest funk I had experienced in my life. My mother had a cake she had baked with the words written on it, "Happy First Date!" I didn't want to spoil her dream, so I told her that we had a terrific time. We sat down and ate the whole thing together.

The next time I saw Bonnie was the first day of classes my senior year of high school. I passed her in the hallway on the way to classes. She said, "Hi." I said, "Hi" back. We really never talked again, and as far as I know, she never mentioned anything to anyone about the amusement park experience. I was very grateful to her for that.

So, between my father dying from being a diabetic, finding out that I, too, had become diabetic, and this very embarrassing first date experience, I surely felt that I had hit bottom. I was going to do something about it. I was going to change. So, I went on one of those starvation diets. I lasted about 4 days until I convinced myself that I didn't want to ride that ride anyway, and there was nothing wrong with being fat.

I didn't realize that I had just lowered the floor for my own personal rock bottom. Now I could sink even lower.

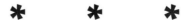

Flash forward to me at forty years old. After years of abusing myself as a diabetic and lowering the floor of my personal bottom to new depths, I finally hit the bottom with a tremendous thud. By this time, food had become my therapist, my friend, my lover. It was probably the thing I thought about most on a day-to-day basis. To counteract this almost criminal intake of food, I started working out at a gym.

One day after finishing on a treadmill, I was getting ready to take a shower. I took off my tennis shoes and saw a little bit of blood on my sock. I took off the sock and discovered a blister about the size of a quarter. I never felt the shoe rubbing against my foot because of a diabetic condition called neuropathy. It deadens the nerves. I have very little feeling in my feet. Blood also does not circulate well down to my feet, which, in turn, makes healing a very big problem.

The blister got worse and worse. I noticed that it was getting very red. I went to the doctor and found out that it was, indeed, infected. They were worried that it might have spread to the bone. In order to contain the infection they would have to arrest it. I asked them directly what they meant by "arrest." They tried to mince their words for a while, but eventually it came down to them discussing the possibility of a partial amputation of my foot. I usually joked around with people. After all, fat people are supposed to be jolly, and that's how I actually made a living—by making people laugh. However, I had no jokes, no wit, and for the first time, no hope.

My timing was right for despair—lunch was about to be served. As I lay in the hospital bed, my friend, my lover, my lunch was just minutes away. If anything could take me away from my problems, it was my meal. In came a smiling face with a food tray. She cheerily asked, "Are you hungry today?" I just told her to slide the food tray on my little stand and back away and that nobody would get hurt. She obeyed politely.

The tray seemed to be filled to the brim with food. It had an enormous plate, covered with a huge plastic dome designed to keep my scrumptious meal warm. I lifted off the plastic dome to witness, much to my surprise (not to mention, dismay), the most measly portion of food I had ever seen. This was the same amount of food I consumed when I took a "taste" of a dish to see if it needs more pepper. I immediately used my nurse-call button to find out what happened to the rest of my food.

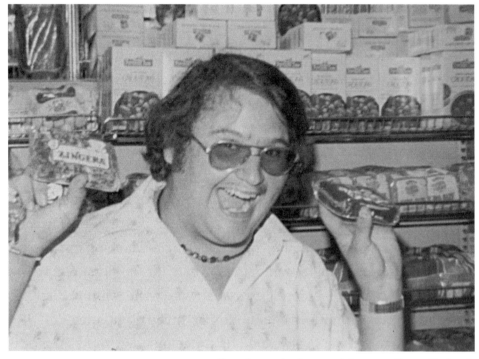

I've always had a special connection with food.

She came over the intercom, "Yes, may I help you?"

"Yes, could you please come in here right away, I have an emergency!"

She and another hospital worker came as promptly as hospital folk do—about 45 minutes later—to ask me what the problem was. I informed them about the missing majority of my lunch. They told me that according to my chart, everything was correct and that I was on a diabetic 800-calorie diet. I was speechless. I immediately got on the phone to my wife and reminded her that she always wanted me to take her on a romantic picnic. "Now's the time!" I told her to bring a picnic basket full of food and let the romance begin.

"You're in the hospital," she stated.

I told her, "Who cares? When I feel romantic, don't question it. Just get up here right away with the basket and don't forget the fried chicken."

She figured me out and refused. I decided maybe this would be a good time to go on a diet. I told myself, "From this point on, I'm on a diet." Then I suddenly realized that the patient in the hospital bed next to me was fast asleep and his non-diabetic, 2500-calorie lunch was staring me in the face. I hobbled out of bed with my sights set on his tapioca. I didn't get more than two steps towards his area when the orderly came in to remove the trays. I slithered back in my bed and tried to distract my hunger with an array of daytime talk shows. 3 o'clock comes around. Dinner is three hours away, there's a repeat of Oprah on TV, and I know I'm not going to be able to withstand watching one more "Poppin' Fresh Dough" commercial. I ring for the nurse again. Over the speaker—before I can say a word—she tells me dinner is at 6 o'clock. I tell her I am no longer hungry, but I need to make some business calls, and I am in definite need of some Yellow Pages. She promptly (45 minutes later) brings me the Yellow Pages, and I immediately start letting my fingers do the walking. As soon as the nurse clears the door, I open the phone book to my favorite Chinese food delivery service.

"One sweet and sour pork, one order of fried wontons, one order of egg-rolls, and some hot and sour soup. Oh, and before you hang up, don't forget the fortune cookies." I told Mr. Lee, "Room 347, bed two."

Mr. Lee gave me a big happy "Okay!" Mr. Lee always seemed happy. No matter what you said to him, he would always reply with a great big happy "Okay!"

I told him, "Whatever you do, DON'T GO TO THE NURSE'S STATION!"

He replied with another big happy "Okay!"

I was satisfied knowing that I would be having a religious experience with my Kung Pao chicken in 30 minutes or less. Awhile later, I saw Mr. Lee roaming the hallway going back and forth carrying my mid-afternoon snack. He went everywhere but my room and eventually ended up at the nurse's station. I guess they called out the big guns then because a nurse I had never seen before—who looked like Lou Cabrazzi from The Godfather and had the personality of Nurse Ratchett—came into my room holding my two bags of Chinese food.

She asked in a big booming voice, "Mr. Furst, did you order this food?"

All I could do was shake my head "No" while fearing this towering creature in a nurse's uniform. About 10 minutes later, someone from the maintenance staff was removing my phone.

Later that afternoon, the same nurse came in to take my blood pressure, and I could smell the fried rice on her breath.

So, here I was…in the hospital waiting to hear if they were going to amputate my foot, while getting caught smuggling in Chinese food. I started to think about the good times in my life. How I wanted to have more good times. I started thinking about my children and how I wanted to see them grow up and dance at their weddings…with both feet. All of a sudden, I felt this tremendous pressure coming from my back. I turned to my side to try to relieve the pain and the pressure. I looked behind me to see if there was anything there that could be causing the pain. Just then I suddenly realized what it was. It was the bottom…I finally had hit bottom.

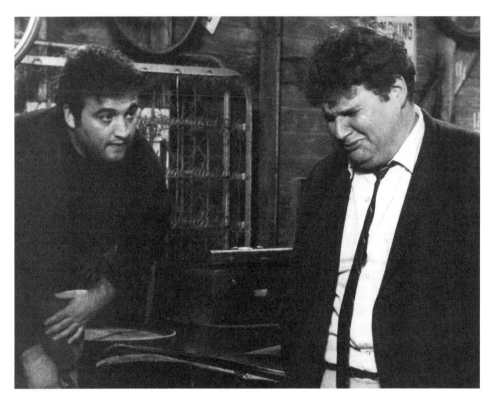

A 1000 calorie diet!? What is a "Flounder" to do? (*Animal House*)

The Nutritionist Was Good Looking

I thought, "I'd like to see my kids grow up. I'd like to see what other movie roles I can get...if I can break into directing," which I have. So I called the nurse and she says, "I'm not ordering food for you." I said that I wanted to see the dietitian. I heard her phone drop. I'd seen the dietitian when she visited the guy next to me. She was pretty—that was motivation, too. She sat and talked with me for about 2 hours and helped me focus on what to change in my diet.

She said, "Oh it's okay, you can eat sugar. It's just another carbohydrate, but if you want to lose weight, it's important not to eat too much fat."

A lot of the stuff I knew. It's common sense. You can eat a lot more vegetables than you can cotton candy. Bring on the veggies. Stay away from the fluffy carbs.

I didn't know there was a difference between white flour and whole wheat flour, because I do love my bagel. You just gotta realize that big bagel you buy has about 60 grams of carb in it!

I think that you can measure your servings for the first week or so, but then you're not going to do that. What I did was take my normal portion, which was for a family of four. And I quartered it! Perfect!

She was very pleasant looking, and I asked her inane questions to keep her there. Anybody that attractive must know what to eat. If I eat what she tells me, will I look as good as she does?

The most important thing I found out was that fat was more important than sugar. She said, "You can eat some sugar, especially natural sugars such as the ones in fruit and milk, but the fat content of your food is important to your weight." I didn't know that about sugar, and I had never looked at the fat content before. When I cut out the fats, the weight started coming off.

She also told me that by losing weight, my own natural insulin would work better, and my diabetes control would be better, too.

After a week on the hospital-imposed 1,000 calorie diet, I came home 12 pounds lighter, and felt good. I said to myself, "I'm going to see if I can continue this." It was an absolute lifestyle change. I never went back to eating the way I had before I hit bottom. It was emotional, it was scary, and evidently, I was ready.

In the hospital, I had combined a huge 32-oz coffee with sugar-free cocoa mix, which would fill me up. That was how I got started inventing recipes to see how much I could fill myself up but with no fat and no sugar. I tried to make my favorite foods without fat—popcorn, potato chips, salad dressing. I looked on the food label and salad dressing has 10 grams of fat per tablespoon. Per tablespoon?! I usually had 9 or 10 tablespoons! One piece of lettuce and 10 tablespoons of salad dressing. Sigh.

Try Breakfast

Before I hit bottom, I don't think I ever ate breakfast, because I ate so much the night before it lasted till lunch the next day. After "Bottom", I'd have a couple of poached eggs, dry toast and, you know, a fruit serving and lots of coffee. Sometimes, I'd have a small toasted bagel with poached eggs. And some fruit and gobs of coffee and be full until 2 or 3 in the afternoon. Or toast a bagel and put lots of sliced tomatoes with salt and pepper on it.

One of my favorite breakfasts is to go to Starbuck's. It would be safe to say that my diet might not be so successful if it weren't for coffee. I just love carbs (bagels and fruit). Carbs and coffee. I'm hyper and happy when I drink a big cup of Starbuck's coffee.

I've spent more than my inheritance at Starbuck's, but I have a comparatively inexpensive homemade breakfast shake. Take 8 ounces of skim milk, add coffee, Equal, and ice. Put it in the blender for a low-fat mocha cappuccino. And it's a lot cheaper than Starbucks. (Don't worry, I do so much business with them they're opening a Starbuck's in my living room next month.)

I would even order what they call a red eye—their full strength coffee with a shot of espresso in it. I'd chug that down, hop in my car, listen to tunes on my radio, and go really fast. About 5 minutes later I'd realize it was only the caffeine, and I hadn't even left the parking space.

Serving Sizes???

I "eyeball" the serving, but weighing out 4 ounces of meat is not for me. In fact, I am notorious for not measuring anything. If I cook something that tastes really good, it's difficult for me to tell you what went in it. I don't organize my kitchen. I just let the creative juices flow. Unfortunately when I get real creative, the juices seem to end up all over the counter and floor. I'll tell you the simple secret to how I cook.

I do know how much one serving of pasta is. I cook that in a pan and then I put in a lot of stuff to make it seem like so much more—lots of onions, mushrooms, peppers. It looks bulky in the bowl, and you fill up when you eat it. I can add chicken or canned clams for a full dinner and feel full—and it's on one serving of pasta. I can add a little Tabasco sauce or curry powder. See? In place of the fat, I spice stuff up. It tastes good. I feel full. And the weight is coming off. Another way is to add a lot of Tabasco to the sauce, which makes you drink a lot of water, which fills you up. I call this the "stupid gringo" diet trick.

Reading the Labels

You need to be careful about eating too many carrots. I didn't know till the dietitian told me that there's sugar in them. I thought I was being healthy. Hey, I'm eating a bag of carrots—they call it diet food, rabbit food. But I didn't realize that my sugar was going up. I ate bags and bags of carrots. I could see better. And it turned my skin orange.

I never read the label for vegetables…but when I eat a serving, it comes in multiples of 12. So I had to do the math. For instance, I would get a box of sugar-free popsicles. They were 15 calories a piece, I'd eat all 12 for less than 200 calories. I got full, but I got a "freeze" headaches.

Another treat was a product like ice cream called Carbo Light. It has like 9 calories per ounce—wow, 20 ounces was 180 calories! My favorites are the blueberry cheesecake and chocolate chip cookie dough flavors.

No Fat, Low Fat

After the hospital, my main goal was to feel as full and uncomfortable as I possibly could—but still lose weight. And that's when I just started to make things up. I would make my own barbecue sauce. I cut out red meat—because I knew it was high in fat. My cholesterol went from 230 to 175 when I lost my weight. Unfortunately, it's back up around 190 now because I'm not trying to lose weight any more.

I would take my homemade barbecue sauce, and I would grill vegetables. I'd brush my homemade sauce on them, so I would have the taste I loved, but no fat. I became a huge fan of the artificial spray Pam and now they've come out with the misto sprayers, so you can put olive oil on your pans. No fat whatsoever.

Actually, I went to an extreme where I cut out all fats—sometimes only eating 3 grams of fat a day—which neither I nor the attractive dietitian recommend that you do. Your body needs the healthy fats that you find in fish, nuts, and olive oil. I love almonds, pecans, and peanuts. (So much so, that I count the serving out and put the container away.) I also eat soy nuts and chop up jicama and munch on the sticks. I usually don't eat anything I can't spell, but I made an exception for jicama (which has no fat, by the way).

Carb Counting

The attractive dietitian also told me about carbohydrate—it makes blood sugar go up. I know a lot of fad diets focus on cutting out carbs, but you need to eat carbs to be healthy. When people with diabetes count carbs, it's to help them control their diabetes. For example, if you eat the same amount of carb at lunch every day, your blood sugar in the afternoon falls into a predictable pattern. I don't really count each carb, but I'm very aware of them. I don't have a problem with not eating sweets. I don't have a problem with not eating fats. I have a problem with "I love carbohydrates." I love bread. I love pasta. I love rice. I got a box of shredded wheat, thinking this is great, no sugar, no fat, no salt—I'll eat the

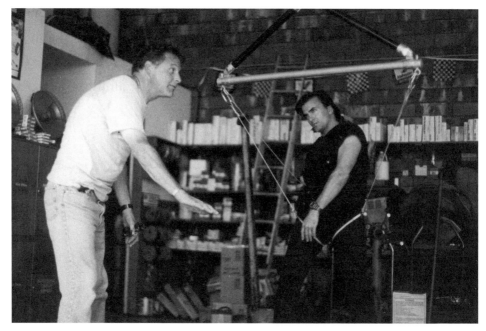

Keeping the energy level up on the set of *D4G* (*Diabetes for Guys*).

whole box! But it was 400 grams of carb! I just found out recently that fruit has carbs! I thought it was like a free food!

I try to watch the carbs, but you know what? Anybody reading this book? I'm not always successful at eating moderate amounts! I love popcorn. I mean, I love popcorn. I don't use oil in the popcorn. I make my microwave movie theater popcorn— which is one of my recipes. And I bring my movie theater popcorn to the movies. Not only do you save EIGHT BUCKS, but it's great popcorn. Later on, you'll see how I use one serving of pasta (carb) with lots of servings of vegetables to make healthier (but still filling) meals.

I'd take the single portion of carb and throw in tons of free food. So I had a gigantic meal, but only the one portion of rice or pasta. And I felt full. And it was low fat and low calorie. This is the opposite of having a little bit of vegetables over a mound of rice. I have a little rice over a mound of vegetables. And lots of spicy flavor.

I'd add chicken, too. I have protein every day, carbs every day. Before I started losing weight, I ate four food groups. I was extremely disappointed when I found out that Reese's pieces was not one of the four. I figured that if ET could eat all these Reese's pieces and not get fat, why can't I?

Chapter Two

An American Childhood

Let me continue with the theme of overeating as an addiction, just like drugs and alcohol. I know that when a drug addict goes to rehab for 30 days, he can't go back to his old ways and his old friends (or even his family if they share the same bad habit). But you can't do that with food. We all have to eat.

I should tell you that I never smoked, never did drugs, never drank alcohol. While other kids in the 70s were smoking pot, I was eating pot roast. I did eat marijuana brownies, but not for the high. In fact, the one time I got extremely high I didn't even know I was doing it. It also has nothing to do with inhaling or not exhaling. I was doing a play in college and at the end of the play's run we had a cast and crew party. Everyone was supposed to bring some food; it was a Potluck Party. Someone must have misunderstood because they actually brought the pot. They had made marijuana brownies, and I have always been a sucker for brownies. I could care less about the marijuana. That night at the party I consumed almost the entire batch, blissfully unaware of its potent ingredients. I had no idea why about an hour later I was having an intimate conversation with my fingers, John Lennon, and Nikita Kruschev all at the same time.

Like most addictions, the food fixation runs in the family. It's very rare that you see overweight kids without overweight parents, too. I have two older sisters, and in my family, we all ate together. We ate together, and we all dieted together. Almost like a contest. I remember having charts on the refrigerator and checking our weight. Then one day one of our charts would be missing... and the diet was gone by the wayside. I was probably eight when I went on my first diet. My parents were thin when they were married but got overweight as time went on.

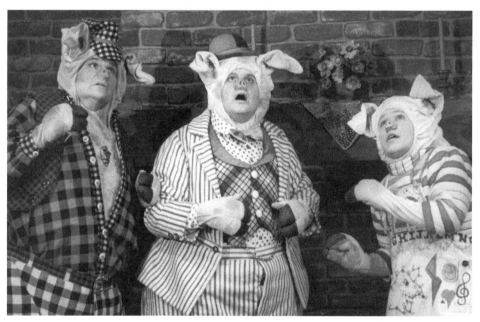

Three Little Pigs...memoirs of my family?
(Showtime, *Fairy Tale Theater.* L to R: Fred Willard, me, and Billy Crystal)

We loved High's Ice Cream stores. We'd stop in for ice cream together. I felt it was my particular job to try every one of their 50 flavors, and I only had 2 1/2 months of summer to do it. We'd discuss what to have for lunch while we were eating breakfast. Our Sunday morning tradition was a trip to an all-you-can-eat buffet. We very rarely sat down at a restaurant where we ordered. I didn't know what a waitress was. To me she was the person you told that the buffet had run out of fried chicken. We weren't wealthy, but we always had money for food. One fat, happy family.

When eating out, my favorite foods were beef and maybe a baked potato, lots of sour cream and butter. We always chose strictly from two starches, potatoes and corn. In TV dinners, I liked the meatloaf dinner because the two veggies were—you guessed it, potatoes and corn! Actually, I always liked the Hungry Man dinner, but I was really waiting for them to come out with the Starving Man dinner. To me, the Hungry Man wasn't realistic. Get a load of the teeny square of dessert! Who are they kidding?

When I was a kid, I went on every diet around. I went on the grapefruit diet. You could eat anything you wanted as long as you ate a grapefruit before it. I scoured every candy store and found grapefruit candy. I gained 50 pounds. I went on a Weight Watchers' diet when I was fourteen. I weighed in at 320 pounds. I was afraid that I'd get too big for the scale—it only went to 350. I didn't want them to have to use the extra counterweight.

I went on OptiFast when I was a teenager...nothing but the milkshake. But I deliberately misread the instructions. In four days I had eaten a month's worth of milkshakes. I told the lady, "I'm never hungry on this diet! And could you give me four more cases of the milkshakes?"

And the Metracal diet. Once again, they had diet dessert for you to eat—Metracal cookies. That was the first time I "accidentally" misread the directions. I didn't really misread the directions, but at the age of 10, I could get away with that. All the Metracal cookies sounded so delicious, but they all tasted the same. The peanut butter ones tasted just like the chocolate mint, and they both tasted like the oatmeal. Well, actually they tasted a little like dog biscuits (but don't ask how I know what dog biscuits taste like. Suffice it to say, I was very hungry that day, and Spot was the only one that would share).

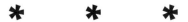

It was terrible that our last name began with an F. As you could guess, we were the "Fat Feuersteins." My nickname in high school was "Marshmallow." It was so accepted. Now I look back on it, and realize the teachers called me that, too. They shouldn't have done that.

I wanted to make fun of myself before someone else did. It didn't hurt as much as it did when someone else did it. In elementary school I was forced to become funny. I made fun of myself because it was better to hear it from me than to hear it from somebody else. That's how I got attention. Not sports, not looks. It was because I was funny. I was sensitive, but I let no one know this. It hurt so much less if I made the jokes.

Like any good addict, my family turned to our addiction to make the pain go away. Eating wasn't a family activity. It was the EVENT. It made us feel good, just like alcohol makes an alcoholic feel good. It numbed any comment a kid might have made. I was always a closet eater, even with my family. I had made a sandwich one time at home and was eating it in the laundry room. I heard my mom coming, so I buried it in the dirty clothes. Throughout the years, my mom probably found enough buried food for the entire cast of *Survival*. And that was just in the whites and linens. (Yeah, I was a closet eater until I was too fat to fit in the closet.)

Then, of course, college came and I was on the meal plan. It was a cafeteria, buffet-style system. I thought I had died and gone to heaven. I was majoring in All You Can Eat 101. Much to my dismay, six months later they started handing out little tickets so you could only go through the line once. They swore that this wasn't because of me. But I started to get a complex anyway.

I always had to shop at the "Big and Tall" man stores, but in all the years I was shopping there, I never once saw a tall man. They were all fat guys just like me. Of course they didn't refer to us as fat guys, we were called portly gentlemen. The only guy who wasn't portly in the store was the salesman, and he looked like something out of GQ magazine. I imagine him going home to his gorgeous girlfriend and telling her about all the fat guys (he was allowed to use the word fat outside of work) he had helped during the day. When I was a kid, I used to hate to shop at the Husky sections of Sears or Penney's. For those of you not familiar with this, the Husky sections were always placed in some obscure part of the store, and you would always have to ask where it was located. I hated shopping back when I was a kid. Vast selections boiled down to the blue pants or the black pants. What I wanted was what everybody else was wearing. I wanted a pair of bellbottoms! My friends were all dressed like they were part of the Monkees, and I wanted to be Mickey Dolenz so bad.

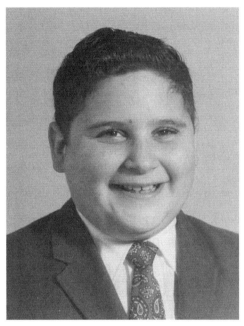

Lookin' stylish at 10 years old.

Unfortunately the Husky section didn't carry bellbottoms. Not even in blue or black. So I bought the blue pants and just pretended to be Mickey. It was a good thing I had a great imagination as a kid, because for a brief moment I did believe I was him. Even if he did appear to be Husky.

One of the steadfast rules of fat person fashion is "never go near corduroy." It's like a cat wearing a bell around its neck. Everyone can hear you coming from miles away. When your legs are too fat, they scrape together, and in corduroy, it sounds like sandpaper being rubbed on a microphone. If you were totally clueless, you'd wear corduroy and horizontal stripes and as you walked down the hall, kids looked like they were in a *Godzilla* movie—hands over their ears as they ran away screaming, unbelievable fear spread across their faces.

The big thing growing up in Virginia Beach was your bathing suit. Speedo was not in my vocabulary. I did go to the beach pretty often, but I stayed away from the whaling boats—in case of mistaken identity. I usually had a good time, but I'm positive I would have had more fun if I had been thinner. I never took anything off; I always wore a big T-shirt over my bathing suit. I even wore the shirt in the water. I always made the excuse of not wanting to get sunburned.

I went to the beach one time with some friends, and we took turns burying each other in the sand. It came time for me to be buried, and they all took shifts. The project was too big to do all at once.

When I was in the Cub Scouts, I was the only one to earn a merit badge for my culinary ability. I took first prize with my wienie toasted marshmallow surprise. When we'd go into the woods, people would snuggle up around the campfire or huddle around me. I thought I had a bunch of friends, but they were just using me for the body heat. During my teenage years I had the typical teenager jobs, but mine would always somehow gravitate towards the food service industry. I remember driving a Mr. Softee ice cream truck one summer. I was called into the

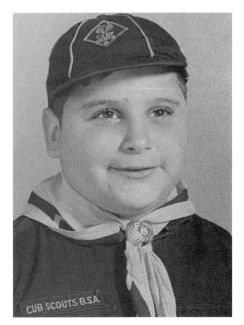

Culinary dreams at age eight.

boss's office because I was moving a lot of product, but my sales weren't up to par. They questioned me about this. Inside I was thinking, "How stupid can you be, just look at me, here's your profits and sales right here," as I gripped the rolls of fat around my midsection. But on the outside I tried to retain my composure. I reminded them about the policy of not charging policeman for ice cream. I asked them if they had seen the news lately. Did they have any idea how high the crime rate had risen and that the streets were swarming with police at all times? Naturally, I felt obliged to offer free ice cream to all of them. The city I lived in wasn't all that big. We may have had about 50 policeman on the entire force back then. Could I get away with telling them that they all wanted seconds?

It's funny, a few years earlier my dad owned an ice cream store but had to close it because it wasn't profitable. I worked there also. I know what you're thinking....

These jobs continued even through college. I drove a truck and worked filling vending machines for Tom's Peanuts. Everyday I was in a truck with bags of peanuts, cookies, chips, and every other snack food known to man, or at least southern Virginia. It was a virtual junk-food smorgasbord on wheels. Okay, so Tom's Peanuts is also no longer in business, but come on, I wasn't *that* hungry.

When I was in college, I was always on a budget, what with my ability to single handedly drive a company under. I could go all day with one meal. Unfortunately, that meal would be a box of Hostess Ho-Ho's and a quart of chocolate milk. With my diabetes, this would make me very ill, and I didn't feel like eating the rest of the day. It worked for the financial plan, but it was making me sick with irreversible effects on my disease.

I think I learned my mindset from my parents. They had terrible eating habits, but, like most kids, I thought they were the greatest and knew everything. So who was I to argue when they put chocolate milk on Sugar Frosted Flakes? Between my parents and my other greatest role model, Tony the Tiger, I was like putty in their hands.

When I was a kid, all my friends decorated their rooms with super hero posters. I did the same, but my heroes were food icons. I had posters of Captain Crunch, The Trix Rabbit, and of course Tony (not Bennett)—Tony the Tiger! I worshipped him. I'd go shopping with my parents, and I'd buy cereals I didn't like because they had the best toys. That was the beginning of the sophisticated food marketing for kids that is leading to rising obesity in children today.

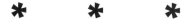

People always ask me, "How did you get your job on *Animal House*?" What is interesting is that every agent in Hollywood turned me down. Even the commercial agents, because they said they don't use fat people in commercials. They don't want fat people hawking food because then people will think they'll get fat if they eat that product.

So I'm in Hollywood, without an agent, and I was delivering pizzas for a restaurant called Two Guys From Italy (and no, I don't know whether they're still in business). It's funny, I never met the second guy from Italy, I only dealt with the other guy from Italy. The restaurant was located in Hollywood, so I would deliver pizza to a lot of stars, producers, directors, and weirdos. I delivered to Carole King and Lindsay Wagner (I had no idea that the Bionic Woman loved anchovies). I even delivered to this rock band named Kiss and got to see them without their make-up—I quickly realized why they wore it. The best part of the job, besides meeting famous people and knowing what kind of toppings they liked on their pizza, was that I got to eat all the stuff that couldn't be delivered because of wrong addresses. It was certainly an adventure, but one I never want to have to go back to.

So what does this have to do with *Animal House*? Well, when I knew I was delivering to a movie person, I would put my picture and resumé in the box with the pizza. I would tape it to the top of the inside flap, so when they opened the box, the first thing they would see was my smiling mug. Hey, don't laugh, it worked. I landed

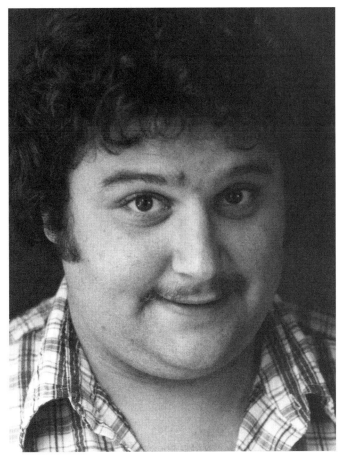

This is my first headshot from when I started out in Hollywood. Picture this on the inside of your pizza box!

an audition for this low budget comedy called *National Lampoon's Animal House*. Three months and six audition call-backs later, I landed the part of the naive freshman Flounder, or as a lot of the critics called me, "the fat, lovable freshman." Hey, there's one time I really didn't mind being called fat. I was starring in a Universal Studios movie!

I did other films after *Animal House*. I was always cast as the fat guy. I mean, what else were they going to cast me as? There aren't a lot of roles written for a 300-pound action hero hunk.

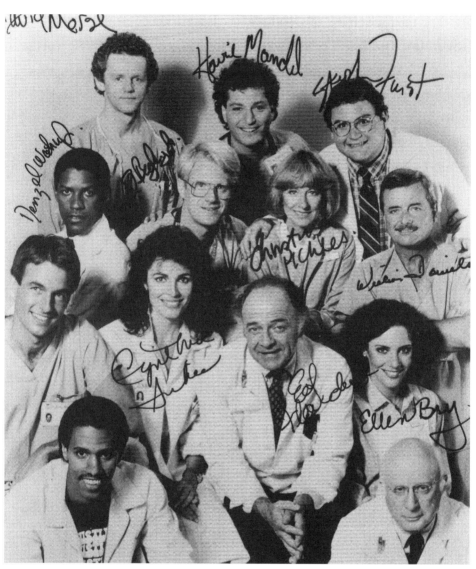

St. Elsewhere © 1983 Twentieth Century Fox Televison.

Several years after *Animal House*, I was cast in the award-winning series *St. Elsewhere*, where I played the fat, naïve, but lovable (no surprise) resident Elliot Axelrod. There were no fat jokes, and it was a serious role in a well-written show with fantastic actors. Actually, the first time I learned a lot about diabetes was on an award-winning episode starring the late Jimmy Coco. He had to get his feet amputated from diabetes complications. I shivered, but told myself that couldn't happen to me.

It's interesting that I never thought I needed to lose weight to be an actor. I remember one day on the set, the executive producer, Bruce Paltrow (Gwyneth's Dad) came down, and during our friendly chat, he asked me about losing weight. I told him how hard it was, that it was like being addicted to food.

He asked me, "An alcoholic can stop drinking. Why can't you stop overeating?"

I told him it is so much easier to stop drinking because you know when you have a problem, and AA says that you can't have any more alcohol—you can quit cold turkey. But three times a day you have to eat to survive. It would be like telling an alcoholic that he can have three beers a day. About 4 weeks later, my character had a scene with an alcoholic where we were arguing over which was harder to kick—an addiction to overeating or to boozing it up. Life imitates art, or is it the other way around?

One thing that has made it easier today than it was when I was dieting as a child and teenager is the large number of lower-fat and lower-calorie foods that are available. I swear I should buy stock in the Equal company. I remember the only product that we had back then was diet soda. Boy, did it taste horrible...full of cyclamates. You remember cyclamates. That's the stuff that made laboratory rats look like the Elephant Man. The soft drinks that I remember were Tab and Fresca. I don't know which tasted worst but, hey, I could drink all that my round Buddha belly would hold, so I got used to it.

We had a special treat whenever my dad returned from a business trip to New York City. There he could buy a special diet soda called No-Cal, which came in exotic flavors like chocolate fudge and coffee. They were like gold. My dad would take an ice cold one, put skim milk in it, and it was terrific! I remember my dad asking me to help unload the car once, and I was bringing out a bag of this "worth-its-weight-in-gold" soda. The bag busted from the bottom, and all the soda broke. The chocolate ones, the coffee ones, even the orange vanilla ones...I thought I was in so much trouble, but my dad came rushing out and saw that my leg was cut. He got upset over my leg, which I hadn't noticed, and I was upset because I thought he was upset about the soda. Once we got it all straightened out and my leg was bandaged up tightly and I'd gotten the hugs and kisses from my mom, we all had a disgusting-tasting Tab to drink.

I remember growing up and being out with my dad, and we would see a really fat person. It became a signature statement of my

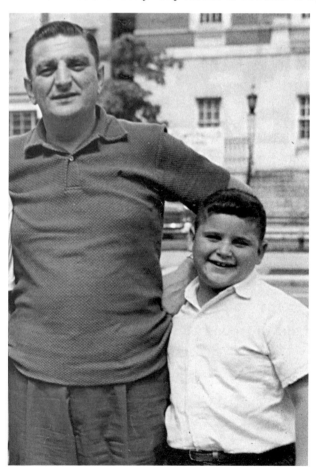

dad's that he would whisper to me, "If you don't stop eating, you'll get as big as that." Even though we were both big, I guess it came as some kind of comfort to us that there was always someone fatter. We were doing just fine being the "right size" overweight. As we tend to parent the way we were parented, I remember saying the same thing to my two boys when they were small and we would see an obese person.

Just the "right size" kind of guys.

But having been that person, and more than likely having been pointed out and whispered about by another parent, I don't say or even think that anymore.

Between me and my two sisters, I was always the thinnest. I took great pride in the fact that when I weighed 320 pounds, I was still the thinnest. I dreaded going back to visit my sisters in Virginia because the natural thing to do was to go out to dinner. I would almost have a mini-anxiety attack right before we would walk into the restaurant because I cared so much what people thought. The stares we would get! I still become uneasy wondering what people were thinking. Were they thinking, "We should order before those 3 fat people order?" Or were they thinking, "My God, I hope they don't seat them next to us because I don't want to lose my appetite." I had an experience like that when Cloris Leachman asked me and actor Stuart Pankin to move to another table because she didn't want to stare at fat people during lunch. This was on the set of a film called *Scavenger Hunt*. Yes, Stuart and I were both fat, but we were extra padded to make us look even fatter than we were.

A lot of times when I was cast in Hollywood, I would always be eating in the scenes. I hated it if it was just for a laugh. I didn't mind eating during a scene if that was what the script called for, but I always hated it when the joke was that I ate more than anyone, or I was stealing food, or I was stuffing my face in a closet. I remember one line in a film I did called *Up The Creek*, and another actor is trying to encourage me to stop eating so much. The line was, "Hey, you got to treat your body right, your body is a temple, but yours is starting to resemble the Houston Astrodome." There were lines like these in a lot of the film and TV work I did over the years. Even though I didn't like it, I was still doing what I had always dreamed of doing, and they were paying me to do it.

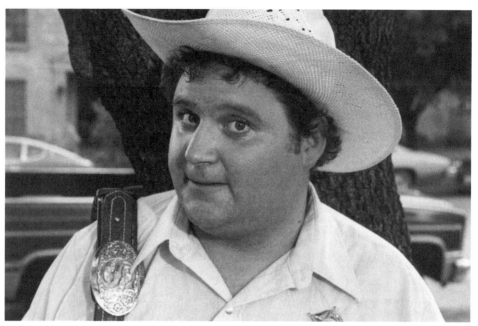
Dreams do come true! An actor and a Cowboy in *Silent Rage*.
(Photo courtesy of Columbia Pictures)

It's like telling a kid who wants to be a cowboy that he can be a cowboy and get paid for it. All I ever wanted to be was an actor or a cowboy. Being a cowboy was the only other job that is probably harder to find work in than being an actor, so I chose to be an actor. Besides, at my size, there were definite drawbacks to riding out on the prairie all day. When was the last time you saw a Burger King out on the prairie?

In *Animal House* I was spoiled. I was in a hit movie, everybody loved my character, and I didn't eat in the entire film. No one even mentioned my weight in the film. Then came the spin-off—a TV show called *Delta House*. The writers quickly resorted to the old Hollywood stereotype of the fat guy eating all the time. Almost every episode had references to my weight, or I was given a food prop to stuff down my throat during a scene. I hated it, but...I was starring in the TV series and being paid nicely. It was either put up with a few fat jokes or go back to delivering pizza. I chose fame and fortune over pepperoni and mushrooms.

My Family

I have always been the main cook in my family. My wife is a vegetarian and after one too many bowls of sprouted wheat grass over sautéed twigs and rice, my sons and I revolted. We ate only the finest corn dogs and kielbasa for a solid week. We didn't even look at anything green. We did have a pistachio ice cream sundae, but I don't really think that counts. I would cook and consume about 1,200 calories in the "taste tests" I conducted to make sure the food was just perfect for my darling children. Sometimes the tasting got carried away, and there wasn't enough for a meal, so we'd end up at McDonald's or Burger King.

Now it's funny because I still am the cook, and everyone likes my stuff, but it's healthy. My kids will say, "This is great, what's in it?" I have to tell them that I don't really know. I just smelled all the various herbs and spices I had on hand and started throwing stuff in. Of course, this drives my wife crazy.

With trying to stay on diets throughout the years, the toughest holiday for me was Halloween. Even back in college it got me into trouble. I remember one Halloween my roommate and I were craving candy real bad, so we donned the sheets from our dorm beds and headed out to the rich neighborhoods where they gave out regular-sized candy bars. Two hours later our pillowcases were filled with our rewards. Unfortunately, we were stopped by the police not long after because some people had reported the KKK marching in the neighborhood. I told them the truth about just being hungry and wanting candy, and they saw what I looked like underneath the sheet. They believed us and let us go Scot-free. Well, I did have to give them some of my candy, but I don't think they considered it a bribe.

Having kids of my own at Halloween was also tough for my various diets—and tough for my kids. Even after all the diets I've been on in my life, I still haven't found one that endorses the consumption of Halloween candy. My kids would come home with big bags of candy loot and the next day, most of it would be mysteriously gone. When they demanded an explanation, I told them we gave it to the poor children. That worked until they saw a bunch of wrappers in the trashcan. They said they had no idea there were so many poor kids living in our kitchen.

I have two sons, and they are as different as night and day—or in my own personal language, as different as a pastrami on rye and a bagel and cream cheese. One is physically fit with a full head of hair; the other is overweight with thinning hair. My older son always complains he got all the bad genes from my wife and me, and his brother got all the good genes. Either way, I am concerned my older son might get diabetes because he's overweight, and they both are susceptible. I know that he can prevent diabetes by losing weight and exercising. But I come from this place where I know that no matter what I say to him, he's got to hit his personal bottom. It might be "Hey, these pants are too tight, and I want to lose some weight." That could be a personal bottom. Or maybe he's got to be diagnosed with diabetes and start having complications. Recently he got engaged and has been losing weight because he wants to look good at his wedding. He is doing it for himself. I didn't say a word because I knew he wouldn't do anything about it until *HE* wanted to. I am extremely happy for him and encourage him all the way. If he falters, I won't say a word, except to continue my encouragement for him when he starts up again.

Diets?

I was never able to stay on a diet because I hated the feeling of being hungry. Who doesn't? When your belly is full, you are content and you feel secure. So when I would feel any insecurity, I would eat. Food was everything to me. My best friend, my lover, my therapist, and my silent buddy all rolled up into one. I have had some great conversations with food. Food actually talks to me. (I consider myself the Dr. Doolittle of food.)

The diet that finally worked for me after all these years was successful because it was tailor-made to me. It wasn't something unnatural to me, like eating 50 grapefruits and nothing else, or the Atkins diet where I couldn't have an apple, but could have a pound of bacon. My diet was food I liked, and I ate until I was full. I had plenty to eat.

I lost weight at a rate of about 2 pounds a week. I have had overweight people come up to me and say that 2 pounds a week seems like it would take an eternity. They say, "If I only lose 2 pounds a week, it will take me a year to lose all the weight I should lose."

I just say that I have never known time to stand still. A year is going to come along anyway, whether they lose weight or not. A year from now they could be having the same conversation, saying they have a year's worth of weight to lose. Or they can be saying, "When are we going to hit the beach, I want to show off my new bathing suit!"

For many years, I would eat and feel bad and guilty about it. And then drown my sorrows by eating again. Food was a comfort to me when I was depressed. I would eat to celebrate some good news. I would eat to drown my sorrow about bad news. If I didn't get something that I wanted, or didn't achieve something, I'd think, "At least I've got this hamburger. I can eat it, and then I'll feel better." And I did feel better. But, it was a superficial bandage, and more often than not, the bad food made me feel worse, which made me depressed, which made me want to eat another hamburger, which…well, you get the picture. I feel so much better when I eat healthfully. When I'd start a new diet I used to say, "God, I feel so much better!"

When I wasn't eating well, I would have 3 diet sodas with a meal. So, I always knew when my blood sugar was under control because I didn't even want to finish one can of diet cola. I would think, "Wow, that's weird." I drink a lot of liquids now (not colas) because they suppress my appetite, and it's an oral thing. There's something I've heard along the way and it's true—if you drink a glass of water before your meals, or start off your meal with some kind of low-fat soup, it fills you up. I can go in thinking I'm starving, but after having a couple of cups of coffee before the meal comes, I'll find I can't finish my meal.

Before hitting bottom, I was always on the "Monday" diet, meaning I was going to start my diet on Monday. (This is similar to the "Tomorrow" diet, which is always starting tomorrow. "Oh,

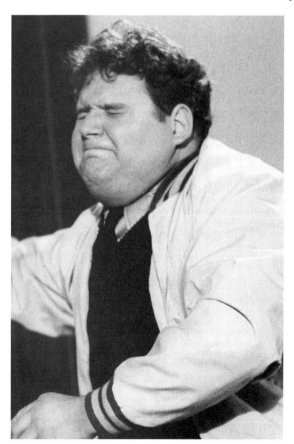

Sunday is so far away! (*Animal House*)

it's okay to eat this 4-pound brick of fried beef, I'm starting my diet tomorrow." But somehow, the "Tomorrow" diet never turns into the "Today" diet.) On the "Monday" diet, Sunday night was my pig-out night. And by Tuesday, I was looking forward to Sunday night again. But once I started the diet that worked, I never let myself get hungry. I'd stop at Starbuck's (thank God, they've opened up one on every corner) and get some caffeine. I don't drink the double mocha frappuccinos—which I think have enough calories to nourish a small country—just coffee. I must admit, though, the one thing I couldn't give up was half-and-half cream in my coffee.

On my diet, I'd have a large coffee and a baguette at one of the various Starbuck's on my block almost every morning. They have a bakery that does a sourdough baguette. It has 110 calories, no sugar, no fat, and it's hard and chewy. I'd eat this baguette and drink the coffee, and I was good to go till 2:00 in the afternoon.

I try to eat a little bit of everything—peanut butter, fruit, pasta—otherwise my body reacts badly. I just can't go on an extreme diet that leaves out lots of foods. But I knew that some tastes had to change. I've learned that my cheesecake recipe doesn't taste as good as Sara Lee's but it's better for me. I have not had a real Sara Lee's Cheesecake in the past 5 years.

I've also learned that I'm human, and I'm going to slide on my diet every once in awhile. This helped me stick with it, because I never let a little slip destroy the whole thing and make me go back to my deadly habits. I have basically stayed with my new lifestyle for the past 6 years, though I haven't been the patron saint of good nutrition 24/7. But, no matter what, I always got back on the diet horse and rode off into the sunset.

For example, I recently found myself in the city of New Orleans, where it was very difficult for me not to falter. Well, everything in New Orleans is fried, battered, sugared, or drenched in sauces. I love spicy foods and Cajun was the name of the game in New Orleans. I went to a casino near my hotel and even the blackjack tables had fried Cajun peanuts. And get this— they were FREE! They were all you could eat, or in my case, all you could eat as well as stuff into your pockets. Just when I thought it couldn't get any worse, the hotel intercom announced that their world famous Cajun buffet was about to open. I crushed, I crumpled, I cracked, I ran to be first in line. Several hours later I was asked to leave when the kitchen staff wanted to go home to their families.

I felt awful the next day, but I started back on my old ways of eating healthy and didn't let that one (even though it was a big one) relapse make me give up everything I had worked for. There's the mystery. Once I started, I never had the desire to go off my diet. I felt so good. I'm not hungry. I thought to myself, "Why didn't I do this earlier?"

Diabetes and Dieting?

I think one of the main reasons I ignored my diabetes for so long was because there were no immediate side effects. I felt tired and thirsty if I ate badly, but if I just waited a few hours, I would back to my old self again. I had no idea what this was doing to my body—but I was ravaging it. I had a doctor tell me once that I was committing slow suicide. He said, "Instead of putting a gun to your head and pulling the trigger, you're taking whacks at your body, damaging a little piece at a time."

Of course I felt he was just being overly dramatic, until years later when I had to have an appointment with a prosthesis maker to see what kind of foot he could make for me. Luckily, that ulcer healed, and I never had to sell all my left shoes.

I always hated those testimonials on TV from the woman who lost 80 pounds on some diet product. The commercials always end with the actress saying, "If I can do it, you can do it." How the hell does she know what I can and cannot do? Does she have my obsession for peanut butter on graham crackers with whipped cream? That is why I never tell anyone, "If I can do it, you can do it." Each person can do it when he or she decides to it for himself or herself. Not for a spouse or a partner or to be able to impress someone. We do it for ourselves when we have decided that we have hit our absolute bottom.

It's Just Common Sense

I think other people, as well as the diet companies, try to make us think that dieting is some kind of mysterious complicated thing. They create entire systems to pretty much starve you—and I've tried them all. I went on the one where you were supposed to eat their "candy" bar instead of a meal. I have been on the ones where you eat cookies instead of a meal or drink a glass of this miracle drink and lose weight. I even went on the severe Optifast diet at UCLA, which lasted about a day and a half. I couldn't believe how hungry I was. The thing is, it doesn't matter what you're eating if you're eating this little. If I only ate a Snickers bar instead of a meal, or drank a McDonald's shake instead of eating

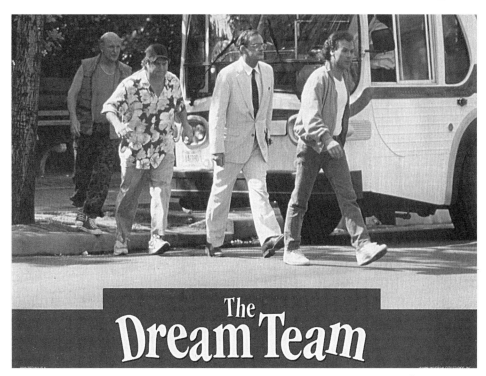

Eating healthy is so simple even these guys could figure it out!
(From L to R: Peter Boyle, me, Christopher Lloyd, and Michael Keaton)

a meal, then I'd lose weight—1,000 calories a day is 1,000 calories a day, whether you're getting it from Slimfast or Ronald McDonald. My problem is that I would drink the Slimfast shake along with a hamburger or eat the whole box of "slim" cookies as a dessert for my regular meal. I was dieting in reverse.

To me it all boils down to common sense. I believe most people know the difference between healthy foods and not-so-healthy foods. Let's see if you can take Stephen's "how-stupid-can-it-be common sense eating test."

1. **What is the healthiest choice of food items in this list?**
   a. A tablespoon of butter
   b. A tablespoon of lard
   c. A tablespoon of olive oil
   d. A tablespoon of Mrs. Butterworth's syrup

I trust that all of you who have read the book to this point picked "c" as the healthiest choice.

2. **Which cereal would you pick for breakfast?**
   a. Captain Crunch with Crunch Berries
   b. Honey Nut Bunches of O's
   c. Lucky Charms
   d. Puffed Rice, Wheat, and Corn combination

It's "a," right? Just kidding. If you picked "d," you've chosen right and gone for whole-grain nutrition and fiber over sugar and heavily processed foods.

3. **One last question, and this will be the trickiest. Which meat dish is the healthiest to eat?**
   a. Stuffed pork chops
   b. Meatloaf with tomato sauce and cheese
   c. Kentucky Fried Chicken
   d. Broiled Salmon with a fruit and chile salsa

If you chose "d," I think you have graduated with honors from the common sense course of sensible eating.

I've been on every insane diet you can possibly imagine. I was on the cabbage soup diet and the only thing I got was gas. I was on the diet where you can eat as much fat as you want, but no carbs. Is that what I am going to do? Let me have a pound of bacon but hold the dry toast? People say, "Well, I can eat as much bacon as I want." I say sure, eat as much bacon as you like, but keep the portable defibrillators close by! We all know what's good for us. We all know what's bad for us. It's common sense.

Eating Styles and Diabetes Control

One of my main problems even today is that I don't eat frequent smaller meals. Just the words "smaller meals" don't seem to fit into my personality. When I'm busy, I can go almost all day without eating. In the olden days, that would leave me so hungry I would eat everything in sight before I went to bed. There was a line in *Animal House* about John Belushi that I think applies to me when I come home at night after not having eaten during the day: "Keep your arms and legs away from his mouth, and it'll be safe."

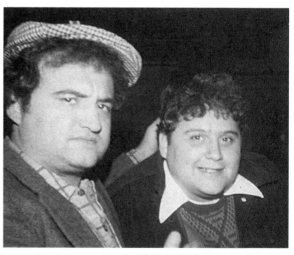
On the set of *Animal House* with John Belushi.

After not eating all day, I was ravenous. This was a terrible lifestyle for someone with diabetes. I was consuming all my calories at one enormous meal at night before I went to sleep. I would even ask, "How can I be fat? I only eat one meal a day." It lasted about 8 hours, but it was only one meal. I remember the old saying, "Eat breakfast like a king and dinner like a pauper." I kind of got it mixed up. I ate breakfast like a king and dinner like the rest of the kingdom. This plays havoc with your blood sugar, which shoots up after a huge meal.

And There Was A1C

I knew a little bit about diabetes from my father, and when I first got diagnosed, I was handed 19,743 pamphlets on how to take care of myself. However, it was all in medical terms. I was saying to myself, "My God, what does urinalysis mean?" At that time I was taking a little yellow piece of paper and dipping it in urine to check my sugar. There were no blood glucose monitors. It was a guessing sort of thing. Oh, what color does this look like? I remember my dad buying test tape. I remember the doctors did it, too. I also remember thinking that if I mixed water in with the urine that the tape would stay yellow. I tried bringing in my touched-up tape to the doctor, saying "Look, it's okay."

What can I say, I was sneaky, but, I learned that you can't trick the A1C. When they ran my first A1C blood test, I tried fasting before the test to get my blood sugar into healthy ranges. My doctor came out and said, "I'm confused. Your blood sugar is 61 but your A1C is 9. That means that your average blood sugar is about 270!" They figured me out.

I didn't want to know about diabetes. I buried my head in the sand. If I don't know about it, it can't happen. It's like saying, "I can't be overdrawn, I've still got checks in my checkbook." But sooner or later I had to face up to it, and unfortunately, it wasn't on my own terms.

Chapter Three

Dessert First

As a child, I would always want to eat my dessert first. I'd eat that and then tackle the meal in hopes that when it came time to get dessert, they would forget I had already had mine. I was also under the impression that if you took just a sliver of cake at a time, it didn't contain any calories. Even if the slivers added up to an entire cake, it didn't count. Those were the rules according to Steve. I rather liked those rules. Unfortunately, my diabetes didn't play by the same rules.

The Cheesecake Caper

When I was about 19 or 20 years old, I was invited over to a college buddy's parents' house for dinner. I was really looking forward to it. The food at college was terrible, but it was all-you-could-eat. Besides, it was very seldom that I was invited over to anyone's house for dinner. I just attributed that to the "fear factor"—the fear other people had about inviting me to a dinner party because then there wouldn't be enough food for anyone else. I, myself, had my own fear factor. I feared being served a normal-sized dinner with no built-in seconds. In other words, the most dreaded phrase for me back then was "portion controlled." I had my own secret weapon that was pretty simple for combating this. I would eat before I went to the dinner. Not only would

I be able to eat like a normal person at the dinner, but I wouldn't be tempted to steal food off someone else's plate while they weren't looking. I could also exclaim with everyone else how stuffed I was from the dinner and truly mean it.

So I had my schedule down: 5 o'clock, shower and dress; 5:45, go to the market and pick up some flowers for the mom who invited me to the "portion-controlled" dinner; 6:05, head for the drive-through window at McDonald's on Franklin Avenue, and then pull up in front of their house at exactly 6:30, just in time for hors d'oeuvres. I just love those little hot dogs wrapped in biscuit dough.

Dinner went off without a hitch. I only had one of everything. Oh, okay, I asked for a second roll, but other than that, I was perfect. Between the McDonald's "appetizer" and the meal, I was truly stuffed. It was then that I heard the best word in the culinary world: CHEESECAKE. I was going to have cheesecake for dessert! I shouted out without thinking, "I'll have seconds! I mean, I'll have some. But just a sliver for me." Darn it. Why did she have to be so obedient? A sliver was all she gave me. But, boy, was that sliver delicious. It was all I could do not to lick the plate. Another person sitting across from me got this enormous piece of cheesecake and then had the nerve to leave a third of it untouched! How dare she? Doesn't she know there are starving children in Africa, or a 300-pound guy sitting next to her that could use that food? To put more salt on this cheesecake wound of mine, when they cleared the table, they put other dishes on top of the unfinished dessert. I was, for once in my life, hoping that they would ask me to help with the dishes, so I could have one last shot at that blatant waste of food. No such luck—they had a maid!

I asked the hostess where she got such a delicious cheese-cake. She said she had to confess that it was just from the supermarket. "It's a Sara Lee strawberry topping cheesecake." I immediately asked if I could borrow a pen and paper to write down this information. After that I made a quick exit. I thanked everyone hurriedly, sprinted to my car, and headed for the nearest late-night market. There it was. It was like staring at the crown jewels. I made my purchase and headed home.

The drive home seemed a lot longer than it did going. Inside my dorm, while other college buddies had their girlfriends over, I had my beautiful Sara Lee. I opened the package and much to my dismay, the cheesecake was still frozen solid. "What do to, what to do?!" I felt like that old Tom and Jerry cartoon where Tom has a can of tuna and no can opener. But not to worry; when it came to food, I had a plan for any obstacle.

I rushed to the common kitchen in the building. I would just defrost the cheesecake a little in the microwave. I closed the door and put it in for two minutes. "That should do the trick," I thought. Those two minutes seemed even longer than the drive home. I could see my cheesecake turning around in the vibrating box. The bell finally dinged! The whole cheesecake was mine! Not just a sliver, but the whole damn thing!!!!

I opened the door of the appliance and took out what was once a beautiful strawberry topped Sara Lee cheesecake. It appeared now to be some kind of cheese soup. It had been completely metamorphosed by the microwave. I didn't realize how much hatred a human could have for a piece of machinery. But to the determined, this was just another small obstacle. I knew I could conquer it. I got a nice napkin and a large soup spoon from the drawer and had a semi-religious experience with my cheesecake, despite its current form. If only I could have been outside my body looking in. A very large fellow, sitting all alone on a Saturday night, eating a melted cheesecake like a bowl of soup. Indeed, a sight to see.

If You're My Friend, Don't Make Me Eat It

People say, "Come on just take one bite. It took me three hours to make this dessert." Yes, and it'll take me 3 seconds to eat it. You'd never say that to an alcoholic—have just one glass of wine—so don't do it to people who are trying to lose weight.

It's so hard to lose weight, and it's so painful. There is nothing about the process that you can hide. There's this huge humiliation factor about being overweight. I saw people looking at me all the time. It was a traumatic experience for me just to go to the beach or a pool. A lot of overweight people try to ignore it, and I did too, but we know it's there. It's hard enough to lose weight, and then you have to do all the psychological stuff, too. We judge ourselves by how others see us. If you're going to lose weight, you're going to need to be on your own side. Start liking yourself. This is hard work you're doing here!

Overweight people are also discriminated against. They did a study where two people go in for a job—one's overweight and the other is not. And 13 out of 15 times, the thin person got the job. People think that being overweight is a weakness. People consider you weak—that you have no will power, that you're not strong. They think that if you can't take care of your own body, how can you take care of business here in the workplace? It's not true. You are not weak. And you can take care of business at work and at home.

So the next time your friends insist you try their homemade turtle cheesecake or their special recipe for chicken fried steak, remind them that what you're doing is tough. No offense to their unbelievably delicious looking meals, but what you need is support, not temptation.

A Note on the Recipes

10% Inspiration, 20% Perspiration, and 70% Using Your Imagination

Dieting is kind of like sex. It's 99 % in your brain—thoughts in your head. Try to think that this cheesecake tastes exactly like the carrot cheesecake at The Cheesecake Factory, and well, maybe it does, a little bit.

A lot of the recipes in this book build on this theory, that imagination can overcome physical reality. I used imagination to come up with a lot of substitutes to my all-time favorites that were better for my body than the fatty originals. Then I'd use even more imagination to pretend that they *were* the real thing. Sometimes my substitutes took a lot of imagination; sometimes they were actually pretty close.

So, as you look through the recipes here, keep in mind that some of the recipe titles might be a little misleading. For example, my recipe for a cheese danish isn't going to taste exactly like a cheese danish. But it's pretty close, and a little positive thinking gets it even closer. Eventually, if you're like me, you'll end up liking these as they are—without the fat, but with lots of flavor.

Imagination Cheesecake

Serving Size, 1/6 of recipe   **Total Servings, 6**

3 egg whites
1/2 cup flour
1 Tbsp vanilla extract
1 tsp baking powder
3/4 cup nonfat milk
30 packets of Nutra-sweet
1/2 cup soft tofu
2 Tbsp wheat germ
1 empty Sara Lee cheesecake box

1. Mix all ingredients together except for the last 2—the wheat germ and empty box.

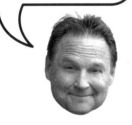

Here is a low-sugar, low-fat recipe I made up for myself so I could keep enjoying one of my biggest weaknesses in the world: cheesecake!

2. Take a pie tin and spray it with butter-flavored nonstick cooking spray. Sprinkle the wheat germ evenly over the bottom of the pie tin. Pour cheesecake mixture over the wheat germ. Bake for approximately 55–65 minutes at 350° F.

3. Let stand for at least 2 hours. Carefully slip finished cheesecake into empty Sara Lee box and refrigerate. DO NOT FREEZE!!!

4. You can experiment with other flavors by adding lemon extract or cinnamon to the cheesecake, or top the whole thing with all-fruit spread.

Exchanges
1 Carbohydrate

Calories 91		**Sodium** . . . . 104 mg	
Calories from Fat. 9		**Carbohydrate**. . . . . . . 14 g	
Total Fat . . . . 1 g		Dietary Fiber . . . . 0 g	
Saturated Fat . . . . 0 g		Sugars . . . . 8 g	
Cholesterol . . . . 1 mg		**Protein**. . . . . 5 g	

Cheese Danish

Serving Size, 1 Danish   Total Servings, 1

1/2 cup nonfat cottage cheese
1 tsp vanilla extract
1/2 tsp cinnamon
2 packets Equal
1–2 slices whole-wheat bread
1 cup fruit *(optional)*

1. Mix all the ingredients together, except for bread and fruit.

2. Toast the bread and spread the mixture on it—use 2 pieces of toast if you want.

3. Bake it in the oven till warm through.

4. You can put 1 cup of fresh raspberries or any fruit you want on top.

Exchanges
2 Starch
2 Very lean meat
1 Fruit

Calories 301		**Sodium** . . . . 706 mg	
Calories from Fat 28		**Carbohydrate** . . . . 48 g	
Total Fat . . . . 3 g		Dietary Fiber . . . . . . 13 g	
Saturated Fat . . . . 0 g		Sugars . . . . 13 g	
Cholesterol . . . . 6 mg		**Protein** . . . . 21 g	

Pudding for Eight (but you can eat the whole thing)

Serving Size, Entire recipe   Total Servings, 1

1 pkg unflavored gelatin
1 serving nonfat dry milk
Flavoring—vanilla, chocolate, pineapple, or whatever you like

1. Put all the ingredients in the blender.

2. Boil the amount of water in the gelatin directions. Pour the water in the blender. Turn it on. When all is mixed, add crushed ice (already crushed) (by you) (exercise).

3. Pour the mixture into a bowl and put it into the freezer for 5 minutes. When it's thickened, remove it. Take a large spoon, and make a big pig of yourself.

4. You can add frozen fruit—strawberries, blueberries—or add diet Swiss Miss or any flavor you want.

Exchanges
Free food

Calories 23	Sodium . . . . 22 mg
Calories from Fat. 0	Carbohydrate. . . . . . . 2 g
Total Fat . . . . 0 g	Dietary Fiber . . . . 0 g
Saturated Fat . . . . 0 g	Sugars . . . . 2 g
Cholesterol . . . . 1 mg	Protein. . . . . 4 g

Baked Apples

Serving Size, 1/4 of recipe   **Total Servings, 4**

4 medium apples
1 12 oz can diet ginger ale
1 Tbsp pumpkin pie spice
10–14 packets of Equal *(or to taste)*
8 oz nonfat plain yogurt *(optional)*
1 tsp vanilla extract *(optional)*

1. Core the apples—using either Red Delicious or for a more tart taste, Granny Smith. Place in baking pan.

2. Pour diet ginger ale in them until it seeps out in the pan. Sprinkle them with pumpkin pie spice and 10 packets Equal.

3. Bake at 300° F for about an hour. When I serve the apple, I fill the hole with nonfat yogurt. I mix the yogurt with Equal (about 4 packets) and vanilla extract.

Don't be fooled by dishes that sound like vegetables. Zucchini bread, carrot cake, fried zucchini sticks...these don't count as part of the 5 vegetables and fruits you should have each day. But this recipe does!

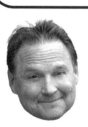

Exchanges
2 Carbohydrate

Calories. 142		**Sodium** . . . . 65 mg	
Calories from Fat. 6		**Carbohydrate**. . . . . . . 32 g	
Total Fat . . . . 1 g		Dietary Fiber . . . . 4 g	
Saturated Fat . . . . 0 g		Sugars . . . . 27 g	
Cholesterol . . . . 1 mg		**Protein**. . . . . 3 g	

Parfait

Serving Size, 1/8 of recipe   **Total Servings, 8**

1 pkg Jell-O brand gelatin *(diet raspberry)*
1 pkg chocolate fat-free, sugar-free Jell-O brand pudding
2 cups fat-free milk *(for pudding)*
16 Tbsp Cool Whip Free

1. Make the gelatin and jell it in the refrigerator.

2. Make the pudding and cool it in the refrigerator.

3. Using a parfait glass, make layers with Jell-O and pudding, about 3 or 4 times. This should fill about 8 parfait glasses.

4. Top each glass with about 2 Tbsp Cool Whip Free.

Exchanges
1 Carbohydrate

Calories 58
  Calories from Fat. 1
Total Fat . . . . 0 g
  Saturated Fat . . . . 0 g
Cholesterol . . . . 1 mg

Sodium . . . . 121 mg
Carbohydrate. . . . . . . 10 g
  Dietary Fiber . . . . 1 g
  Sugars . . . . 4 g
Protein. . . . . 3 g

Summertime Popsicles

Serving Size, 1/4 of recipe   Total Servings, 4

1 pkg chocolate fat-free, sugar-free Jell-O brand pudding
2 cups fat-free milk *(for pudding)*
1 small banana cut in quarters, or 4 fat strawberries
4 Dixie cups

1. Make pudding as directed, using fat free milk.

2. Put fruit in Dixie cups. You can insert wooden popsicle sticks if you have them.

3. Fill with Jell-O pudding and freeze.

4. Peel off the cup, and you have a great popsicle.

Exchanges
1 Carbohydrate

Calories 95		**Sodium** . . . . 176 mg	
Calories from Fat. 2		**Carbohydrate**. . . . . . . 18 g	
Total Fat . . . . 0 g		Dietary Fiber . . . . 1 g	
Saturated Fat . . . . 0 g		Sugars . . . . 8 g	
Cholesterol . . . . 2 mg		**Protein**. . . . . 5 g	

Lemon Birthday Cake

Serving Size, 1/12th recipe   **Total Servings, 12**

8oz fat-free cream cheese
10 packets Equal
1/2 tsp lemon extract
4 egg whites
1-1/2 cups nonfat milk
3 cups flour
1 Tbsp baking powder
2 containers Crystal Light drink mix *(lemonade flavor)*
1/2 cup Smuckers Light apricot preserves
Sugar-free birthday candles

1. Let cream cheese soften at room temperature. Mix cream cheese with about 10 packets of Equal and lemon extract. This will serve as your icing, set it aside.

2. In a separate container, beat egg whites and milk together, add all dry ingredients, and mix.

3. Spray a generous portion of yummy butter-flavored Pam on two 8-inch round cake pans. Pour batter evenly into the two pans. Bake at 350° F for about 20 minutes.

4. Take cakes out of oven using oven mitts (I can tell you from experience that the mitts are necessary!). Cool on a wire rack.

5. Place 1 cake topside down on a cake plate, and spread a thin layer of cream cheese mixture on top. Then spread a thin layer of the preserves on top of the cream cheese. Place the other cake on top and spread the rest of the cream cheese icing on the whole cake.

Exchanges
2 Carbohydrate

Calories. 174	**Sodium** . . . . 226 mg
Calories from Fat. 3	**Carbohydrate**. . . . . . . 33 g
Total Fat . . . . 0 g	Dietary Fiber . . . . 1 g
Saturated Fat . . . . 0 g	Sugars . . . . 7 g
Cholesterol . . . . 3 mg	**Protein**. . . . . 8 g

Lemon Poppy Seed Muffin Bread

Serving Size, 1/15 of recipe   Total Servings, 15

3 cups all purpose flour
1 Tbsp of baking powder
30 packets of Equal
1 tub of Crystal Light drink mix *(lemonade flavor)*
1/2 cup of poppy seeds
1 egg
3 additional egg whites
1 Tbsp Canola oil
1 cup of water

1. Mix all ingredients together and pour into a 9 x 9 pan that's been sprayed with butter flavor cooking spray.

2. Bake for about 30 minutes at 350° F in a square pan.

3. Cut into squares and eat with a great cup of Starbuck's coffee, or sell it at your workplace.

Exchanges
1 1/2 Starch
1/2 Fat

Calories. 142		**Sodium** . . . . 90 mg	
Calories from Fat. 32		**Carbohydrate**. . . . . . . 23 g	
Total Fat . . . . 4 g		Dietary Fiber . . . . 1 g	
Saturated Fat . . . . 0 g		Sugars . . . . 3 g	
Cholesterol . . . . 14 mg		**Protein**. . . . . 5 g	

Chapter Four

Back to the Top: Appetizers

To me, appetizers were created as a way of teasing the appetite. From the unrealistically delicious names, to the tiny portions, to the fact that you're supposed to share with everyone at the table. All I know is that as a fat person, I didn't need any teasing whatsoever. I was always ready and very willing to eat a full-course meal (the more courses the better) without being tantalized.

You know how you have to play food games with little kids so they'll eat their food? When I was growing up, we had food games that were designed to do exactly the opposite. We would all sit around the table, put a piece of chocolate cake in the middle, and see who could withstand the temptation longest. The problem with the game was that each of us didn't care if we lost. As a matter of fact, we all wanted to lose, because the loser got the chocolate cake and the winners just went hungry.

Later on as a young adult, I would have dinner parties. For appetizers I would drape small plates with large lettuce leaves as a background garnish (because as we know, presentation is half the battle of a good dinner), and then serve a small mound—just enough to tease the appetite—of M&Ms mixed with peanut butter. People raved about this appetizer, and even better, there was always a lot left over for me the next day.

As the years went by, food manufacturers made appetizers very easy to serve. They made little frozen delights where all you had to do was pop them in the oven and 10-12 minutes later, you looked like you had slaved in the kitchen all day. Some of my favorites were the jalapeño popovers. These deep-fried little puffs contain jalapeño peppers oozing with melted cheese. Naturally, I found a way to make them even more unhealthy by cooking up a sour cream and ground beef dip to dunk them in.

I also liked the little mini quiches. I'd try to buy them at warehouse stores because they only sell them in bulks of 500, and you were guaranteed to be in quiche heaven for almost a week after any dinner party. The best thing about the mini quiche is the fact that they are called "mini." To me, anything called "mini"—or "light" or "low fat" or even "fat free"—was fair game. You could eat as much as you wanted and, in theory, never gain an ounce of fat. This theory proved to be a little inac-curate once the proof became apparent, and I passed the 300-pound mark on the scale. (And when it comes to diabetes, low-fat foods usually have more carbohydrate than the regular version of the food. A double disaster!)

So, to have a successful gourmet dinner party or just a little appetite teaser for your own meal, I have come up with a few appetizers that are great and good for you, too. Oh, about the peanut butter M&M surprise? After several attempts to try to find a healthy substitute the way I like to do, I realized I couldn't come up with a low-calorie, healthy version. I tried wet wheat germ and green peas with little Ms painted on them, but it just wasn't the same. But if you've really got a hankering, try a couple of bites of the original. Just make sure somebody will take the rest of it away after that.

Crudités (pronounced "crew-de-tays")

Serving Size, 1 Cup veggies & 2 Tbsp dip   Total Servings, 8

8 cups raw vegetables
1 cup fat-free sour cream
1/2 packet dry onion soup mix

1. Cut up your crudités of choice, such as red and green peppers, mushroom, broccoli heads, cauliflower heads, zucchini sticks, carrots, summer squash sticks, etc.

I always loved the sound of this word. It sounds so fancy for "sliced up veggies!"

2. Take the fat-free sour cream and add dry onion soup mix (or vegetable dry dip mix) and put the dip in the center in a hollowed out red pepper. It's fancy, but it's delicious, too.

Exchanges
1/2 Carbohydrate
1 Vegetable

Calories 57		**Sodium** . . . . 219 mg	
Calories from Fat. 3		**Carbohydrate**. . . . . . 12 g	
Total Fat . . . . 0 g		Dietary Fiber . . . . 2 g	
Saturated Fat . . . . 0 g		Sugars . . . . 5 g	
Cholesterol . . . . 2 mg		**Protein**. . . . . 3 g	

Stuffed Mushrooms

Serving Size, 2 Mushrooms   Total Servings, 10

1 lb large mushrooms (about 20)
1/2 cup reduced-fat pepper jack cheese
1/2 cup chopped fresh basil
1 clove minced garlic
1 cup dry bread crumbs

1. Cap the mushrooms and mince the stems in a food processor. Grate the cheese and set aside. Chop basil and mince the garlic. You can use more cloves if you want to.

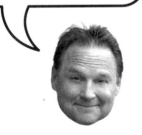

The great thing about this recipe is that you can change the filling ingredients. Sometimes I add crabmeat, ground chicken, spinach, or artichokes.

2. Sauté mushroom stems, basil, and garlic with olive oil cooking spray and a little chicken broth. Add dry bread crumbs and stir till moistened.

3. Add the cheese last and only cook for about a minute. Remove the stuffing from the pan and stuff the mushroom caps.

4. Bake them on a cookie (sigh) sheet for about 10 minutes. Then, broil them for about 2 minutes to crisp the tops. Serve with lemon wedges.

Exchanges
1/2 Starch
1 Vegetable
1/2 Fat

Calories 88	**Sodium** . . . . 141 mg	
Calories from Fat. 19	**Carbohydrate** . . . . 13 g	
Total Fat . . . . 2 g	Dietary Fiber . . . . 2 g	
Saturated Fat . . . . 1 g	Sugars . . . . 2 g	
Cholesterol . . . . 4 mg	**Protein** . . . . 6 g	

Shrimp Cocktail

Serving Size, 1/4 of recipe   Total Servings, 4

16 Jumbo shrimp
1/2 cup cocktail sauce
1 Tbsp lemon juice

1. Buy jumbo shrimp.

2. Boil jumbo shrimp.

3. Mix the cocktail sauce with fresh lemon juice.

4. Think about how incredibly easy this is.

Exchanges
1/2 Carbohydrate
2 Very lean meat

Calories 97		**Sodium** . . . . 456 mg	
Calories from Fat. 10		**Carbohydrate**. . . . . . . 10 g	
Total Fat . . . . 1 g		Dietary Fiber . . . . 1 g	
Saturated Fat . . . . 0 g		Sugars . . . . 7 g	
Cholesterol . . . . 80 mg		**Protein**. . . . . 11 g	

Hummus

Serving Size, 1/8 of recipe   **Total Servings, 8**

1 package dry hummus mix
Lemon juice *(to taste)*
Chili powder, hot sauce, dill *(optional)*

This poor man's version of hummus is great with pita bread, and once you feel you've had a good serving of carbs, you can switch to dipping veggies in it. However, you do get penalized for double dipping.

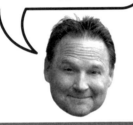

1. Prepare dry hummus mix and add lemon juice and water, depending on how much you really like that lemon taste.

2. I do many, many variations on this dish. In the past I've added extra garlic powder, or added chili powder along with some hot sauce. I've even added dill. You can let your imagination run wild, but that doesn't count for your exercise for the day.

Exchanges
1 Starch

Calories 90	**Sodium** . . . . 314 mg
Calories from Fat. 30	**Carbohydrate**. . . . . . . 12 g
Total Fat . . . . 3 g	Dietary Fiber . . . . 1 g
Saturated Fat . . . . 1 g	Sugars . . . . 0 g
Cholesterol . . . . 0 mg	**Protein**. . . . . 3 g

Nachos

Serving Size, 1/16 of recipe   **Total Servings, 16**

1 16 oz bag baked chips
1-1/2 cups salsa *(p. 73)*
2 oz low-fat or nonfat pepper jack cheese *(grated)*
2 Tbsp chopped jalapeños *(or to taste)*
1/2 tsp chili powder *(or to taste)*
1/2 tsp garlic powder *(or to taste)*
1 can black beans or nonfat refried beans
1 lime, cut into quarters

1. I buy the baked Tostito's chips, which have 1–1/2 grams of fat per serving. I throw them on a plate. (Actually, I don't throw them, but intricately put them into fun designs like the Liberty Bell, replica of the Alamo, Michael Jackson's nose, etc.)

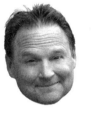

This is one of my favorites because I just love spicy food.

2. On top of the chips, I put the salsa, low-fat or nonfat pepper jack cheese, chopped jalapeños, chili powder, garlic powder, some black or refried nonfat beans, and garnish it all with fresh lime.

3. Pop the layered nachos into the microwave for a minute or two, until the cheese has melted and all is heated through. Serve this and watch your guests just "oooh" and "ahhh" at the great dish. If you have the time and money, you could hire a mariachi band to complete the atmosphere.

4. You can also make fajitas nachos with this recipe by adding some sautéed onions and green and red peppers.

Exchanges
2 Starch

Calories 150		**Sodium** . . . . 382 mg	
Calories from Fat 15		**Carbohydrate** . . . . 30 g	
Total Fat . . . . 2 g		Dietary Fiber . . . . 4 g	
Saturated Fat . . . . 1 g		Sugars . . . . 1 g	
Cholesterol . . . . 3 mg		**Protein** . . . . 6 g	

Stuffed Mini Cabbages with Sweet and Sour Sauce

Serving Size, 1/16 of recipe   Total Servings, 16

1 head green cabbage
1 lb ground turkey
2 garlic cloves, minced
1 tsp dried mint leaves
Salt and pepper *(to taste)*

Don't be fooled by the word "mini" here. They still count as calories. This will take a bit more time but it's well worth it.

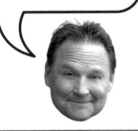

1. You take cabbage leaves and boil them just so they are soft enough to fold around a filling. Cool.

2. Sauté ground turkey with minced garlic. When turkey is browned, add mint, salt, and pepper.

3. Put 2 tablespoons of the filling onto a cabbage leaf and roll up. Cover with sweet and sour sauce, the next recipe!

Exchanges
1 Very lean meat
1 Vegetable

Calories 61	**Sodium** . . . . 336 mg
Calories from Fat. 10	**Carbohydrate**. . . . . 6 g
Total Fat . . . . 1 g	Dietary Fiber . . . . 1 g
Saturated Fat . . . . 0 g	Sugars . . . . 5 g
Cholesterol . . . . 16 mg	**Protein**. . . . . 7 g

Sweet and Sour Sauce

Serving Size, 1/16 of recipe   **Total Servings, 16**

1 46 oz container tomato juice
Juice of 1 lemon
6 packets Equal
1 clove garlic, minced, or...
1/2 tsp garlic powder

1. Put all ingredients into
   a medium-size pan.
   Simmer the mixture
   until it gets thicker.

2. Spoon over rolled
   cabbage leaves and
   bake them in the oven
   at 350° F for about
   15 minutes.

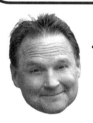

It's just like mama used to make back in Poland. Of course, my mother never stepped foot in Poland, but it sounds more authentic than "just like my mama used to make back in Virginia Beach."

Exchanges
Free food

Calories 18	**Sodium** . . . . 315 mg
Calories from Fat. 1	**Carbohydrate**. . . . . 4 g
Total Fat . . . . 0 g	Dietary Fiber . . . . 0 g
Saturated Fat . . . . 0 g	Sugars . . . . 3 g
Cholesterol . . . . 0 mg	**Protein**. . . . . 1 g

Chapter Five

Beef, Veal, Lamb, and Liver

Growing up I was a big beef eater. I loved hot dogs, hamburger, steak, meatloaf, meatballs, entire hogs…shall I go on or do you get the picture? Other than the "thrill of my life" dating extravaganza with Bonnie, my only other dating experience revolves around a piece of roast beef.

I was on a date, and I was trying to be Mr. Joe Cool. Keep in mind that it's very hard being Mr. Joe Cool when your 2 nicknames are Marshmallow and Stevie Popcorn. Anyway, I was making very good conversation and felt things were going reasonably well when I decided to take a big bite of roast beef—too big a bite. I started to choke and suddenly had a decision to make—shall I remain Joe Cool and just have them give me a simple funeral in the morning, or do I completely embarrass myself and dislodge the side of beef that I so bravely kept trying to swallow. I was only about 18, so I decided to take life over death. At first, I tried to give myself the Heimlich maneuver. Because I had the reputation of being a class clown, my date thought it was just one of my funny routines. But as I started to turn the color of Papa Smurf, she began to realize that even the class clown wouldn't go that far for a laugh. I was eventually able to dislodge the half-eaten piece of beef by groping for it and pulling it out of my mouth. I was also successful at never being able to ask that date out ever again.

I'm a big fan of barbecued foods. I played a character in a movie called *The Unseen* who was locked in the basement. My make-up took 5 hours to apply and had lots of rubber pieces. Any kind of oil or grease would make it come unstuck, so I had to eat through a straw—mostly milkshakes (and not the diet kind, by the way). But one day they had barbecued ribs on the set, and I couldn't stand it. I had to have some. I tried to wipe the grease off, but... there I was, in the middle of a scene, and my rubber lips fell off. They stopped shooting. The director said, "Steve, did you eat the barbecued ribs?" Of course, they could tell. In that make-up, I couldn't see very well and it was all over my costume.

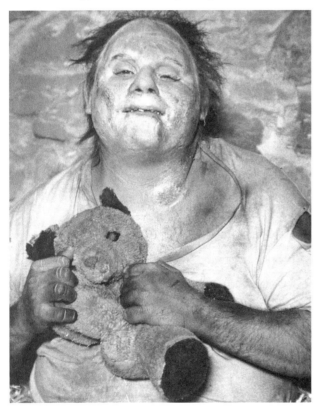

Please, give me some ribs! I'm starving! (*The Unseen*)

Oh, by the way, there aren't any recipes in this chapter. I don't eat beef any more. Or any of those other meats, either.

Chapter Six

Chicken and Seafood and, Um, Condiments?

I love chicken. You can use it almost anywhere, cook it almost any way you can imagine, and make it as healthy as you want. Of course, I'm not the only one who loves chicken. The chicken industry has exploded in the last decade trying to keep up with this country's demand for our fowl friend. Unfortunately, a lot of this chicken is being dropped into batter and a deep fryer before being dropped down our gullets. But when used right, chicken can be very healthy and very tasty.

Seafood is also a great meat for all of us looking to drop those pounds and inches. As far as my seafood recipes go, they're all the same as the ones I use with chicken. I just slide a salmon steak in for the chicken in a barbecue chicken recipe, and I've got a delicious variation.

One of my big downfalls, however, is that I also love condiments—salad dressings, barbecue sauce, mayonnaise, anything. Luckily, I'm pretty label conscious now—I read labels all the time. Back when I started losing weight, I'd read the labels on condiments and they would blow my mind. Is there anything *but* fat in a jar of mayonnaise? They also didn't have all the low-fat substitutes they do now. On my diet, I got to be very mustard friendly. And I learned to make my own ketchup. In this chapter, I've included some of my homemade variations on condiment classics.

I'll Take a Bowl of that Delicious Looking Green Stuff

While we're on the subject of healthy fare, I'll regale you with my tale of how I went from my classic seafood dinner of 4 McDonald's fish fillet sandwiches with extra tartar sauce to becoming the sushi king of southern California. If you've ever eaten sushi, you're familiar with wasabi, that neon green glob of spice plopped on your wooden sushi plank. At first, I thought wasabi was a pistachio pudding. I swore I only wanted a taste and that after my dessert splurge, I'd still continue my diet. I stuck to my guns and was prepared to eat just one tablespoon full of this sinfully rich-looking pudding. It was a heaping spoonful, but it was still just one.

Well, after being rushed to the emergency room for an overdose of wasabi paste, I realized I had just learned a valuable lesson. I immediately gave up the idea of having just one little taste of anything I knew would undermine my new determination. Just like an alcoholic, you can't have just one highball for the holidays.

Chicken Apricot

Serving Size, 1 Chicken breast   Total Servings, 4

1/3 cup apricot jam
1 tsp dehydrated orange peel
4 boneless, skinless chicken breasts (about 1 lb)

1. Mix jam and orange peel together. Set aside.

2. Broil chicken with no spices. There shouldn't be any pink in the meat when it's done. At the last 5 minutes of cooking, remove the chicken from the oven and pour the apricot jam and orange peel mixture over it. This makes a glaze. Return the chicken to the grill or broiler for 2–5 minutes.

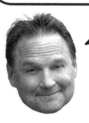

I make a variation with fresh dill. It's called Chicken Apricot Dill. I also make a variation with my salsa and call it Chicken with Salsa.

Exchanges
1 Carbohydrate
4 Very lean meat

Calories. 198	**Sodium** . . . . 71 mg
Calories from Fat. 26	**Carbohydrate**. . . . . . . 17 g
Total Fat . . . . 3 g	Dietary Fiber . . . . 0 g
Saturated Fat . . . . 1 g	Sugars . . . . 13 g
Cholesterol . . . . 68 mg	**Protein**. . . . . 25 g

"Fried" Chicken

Serving Size, 1 Chicken breast   Total Servings, 4

4 boneless, skinless chicken breasts *(about 1 lb)*
1 cup cornflakes or bread crumbs
olive oil spray

1. Wet the chicken breasts.

2. Crush the cornflakes or bread crumbs with a rolling pin or in a food processor.

3. Spray the chicken with olive oil and roll in breadcrumbs.

4. You can also sprinkle on spices and herbs of your choice and bake at 350° F for 45 minutes.

Exchanges
1/2 Starch
4 Very lean meat

Calories. 160		**Sodium** . . . . 134 mg	
Calories from Fat. 26		**Carbohydrate**. . . . . 6 g	
Total Fat . . . . 3 g		Dietary Fiber . . . . 0 g	
Saturated Fat . . . . 1 g		Sugars . . . . 0 g	
Cholesterol . . . . . . 68 mg		**Protein**. . . . . 26 g	

Steve's Ketchup

Serving Size, 2 Tbsp   Total Servings, 30

1 46 oz container tomato juice
10 packets Equal *(or to taste. I use a TON of Equal.)*
1/4 cup vinegar

1. Mix the ingredients in a pan and cook over low heat until it
becomes thick.

Exchanges
Free food

Calories 10   Sodium . . . . 168 mg
  Calories from Fat. 0   **Carbohydrate**. . . . . . . 2 g
Total Fat . . . . 0 g   Dietary Fiber . . . . 0 g
  Saturated Fat . . . . 0 g   Sugars . . . . 2 g
Cholesterol . . . . 0 mg   **Protein**. . . . . 0 g

Steve's Barbecue Sauce

Serving Size, 2 Tbsp   **Total Servings, 30**

1 46 oz container tomato juice
4 packets Equal *(or to taste)*
1/4 cup vinegar
1/4 tsp Liquid Smoke *(or to taste)*
1/2 tsp Tabasco sauce

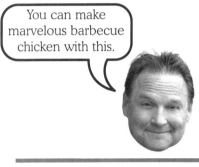

You can make marvelous barbecue chicken with this.

1. To make barbecue sauce, start with tomato juice and add the Equal and vinegar. Put them in a pan and simmer.

2. Then add Liquid Smoke and Tabasco sauce in small amounts to suit your taste buds.

Exchanges
Free food

Calories 9
  Calories from Fat. 0
Total Fat . . . . 0 g
  Saturated Fat . . . . 0 g
Cholesterol . . . . 0 mg

Sodium . . . . 168 mg
Carbohydrate. . . . . . . 2 g
  Dietary Fiber . . . . 0 g
  Sugars . . . . 2 g
Protein. . . . . 0 g

Salsa

Serving Size, 1/4 cup   **Total Servings, 12**

20 oz can chopped tomatoes
1 Tbsp fresh lime juice
1 bunch cilantro, chopped
1 onion, chopped
1 garlic clove, minced
2 packets Equal
1 jalapeño pepper, minced *(don't wipe your eyes!)*
Slices of pineapple or papaya *(optional)*
Baked chips *(with 1.5 grams of fat per serving)*

1. Mix all ingredients from the tomatoes to the jalapeño pepper. You can do it in a food processor if you like.

2. Garnish with a slice of pineapple, papaya, or avocado. Serve with baked chips.

Exchanges
Free food

Calories 17	**Sodium** . . . . 95 mg
Calories from Fat. 1	**Carbohydrate**. . . . . 4 g
Total Fat . . . . 0 g	Dietary Fiber . . . . 1 g
Saturated Fat . . . . 0 g	Sugars . . . . 3 g
Cholesterol . . . . 0 mg	**Protein**. . . . . 1 g

Guacamole

Serving Size, 2 Tbsp   **Total Servings, 12**

1 medium avocado
1/2 cup my salsa

1. Mash up the avocado with my salsa. If necessary, add extra hot sauce to taste. You can also add a little bit of salt and pepper.

Exchanges
1/2 Fat

Calories 30	Sodium . . . . 18 mg	
Calories from Fat. 23	Carbohydrate. . . . . . . 2 g	
Total Fat . . . . 3 g	Dietary Fiber . . . . 1 g	
Saturated Fat . . . . 1 g	Sugars . . . . 1 g	
Cholesterol . . . . 0 mg	**Protein**. . . . . 0 g	

Chapter Seven

Then There's Turkey

Turkey is just about the most low-fat meat product out there, which is great for all of us fighting the battle of the bulge. When I went on my diet, I cut out almost all forms of fat. At the time, I didn't know the difference between good and bad fat and I was eating a total of less than 5 grams of fat a day. While that made me lose weight, it just wasn't healthy.

One night about 3 AM, I felt this tremendous pressure in my chest. I'm thinking, "Oh Great! I'm finally dieting and exercising for the first time in my life, and now I'm going to die of a heart attack." I lay in bed for about 45 minutes, and it didn't go away. So, I drove myself to the hospital expecting an interlude with the defibrillator paddles. I was wrong. They didn't do bypass surgery—they did an emergency gallbladder removal. Immediately after the surgery, I asked the doctor about how much it weighed because I was going to add that amount to my weight loss total. You got to take it wherever you can.

Another problem I had (one that a lot of people of the overeating persuasion seem to have) is the size of the portion. I will read a label and think, "Oh, these cookies have only one gram of fat." Then I realize on closer examination of the Nutrition Facts label that one cookie is somehow 4 servings. Now I ask you, "How many people cut a cookie into fours and split it with their friends?" I don't have friends that I would give 3/4 of my cookie to, anyway.

Recently, I was told I could have a serving of almonds if I wanted to. I got very excited 'till I found out that a serving consisted of 6 almonds. I tend to eat in multiples of 6, so that would make one serving for me 36 almonds. And too much fat—even if it is healthy fat.

When I like something from a restaurant, I always try to duplicate it at home. I did this even before I went on my diet. I had been working for a year to unlock the code of Jack in the Box's secret sauce. It took many months and several hundred burgers to finally figure out that the secret sauce was just mustard and ketchup mixed together. And to make matters worse, after I broke the code, they discontinued the sauce. But I did get to eat all those hamburgers for what I felt was an extremely good cause.

Another secret recipe that I never did figure out was the Colonel's 11 secret herbs and spices. I got it down to 3 secret herbs and 6 secret spices, but even after many buckets of his wonderful tasting fried chicken, I could not come up with the last two secret ingredients. And now, since I have changed my lifestyle, I will probably never find out. Hey, it just dawned on me why the Colonel was so fat. (And it's not a secret.) He's gone, but they've kept him by turning him into a cartoon. I know a bit about life as a cartoon.

Being a fat actor who has suddenly lost a lot of weight changes your image. It does have an effect on one's career. As a human, I started playing different types of roles, and the roles were not as easy to get. People in Hollywood saw me one way for 20 years and didn't really buy me as someone who might actually have a love interest as a character. What's really ironic is that I am still playing obese cartoon characters. I played the fat alien on *Buzz Lightyear and the Star Command*. I played the fat fan-boy on *Freakazoids*. I played the fat walrus on *The Little Mermaid Part 2*, and I played the fat baby elephant on *Jungle Cubs*. I wonder if cartoon characters can have cartoon heart attacks and diabetes complications?

Thanksgiving

I just love holidays. I love all the decorations around the house and the family you get to see and all the gossip about the family members who didn't show up. My favorite holiday of the year is Thanksgiving. Forget all the Christmas presents. Forget the spreading of good cheer. Give me the holiday that is solely based on stuffing your face until you have to be rolled away from the table so you can start the exhausting task of sitting in front of the TV watching football all day (or the *Twilight Zone* marathon). When I was on my diet, Thanksgiving was one of the hardest holidays to conquer. The only thing I could still eat from the fat days was turkey and then I wasn't able to eat the best part—the crispy, fatty skin. I remember the first Thanksgiving I cooked two completely different dinners. One with all the fat and trimmings and one with all the trimmings, but no fat. Most of the people in attendance could not tell the difference between the two dishes, and if they could, they seemed to like the lower-fat, healthier dish instead.

The following are a few Thanksgiving recipes to help you through my favorite holiday. Set your dishes alongside the skinny people's side dishes and appetizers, such as that special artichoke dip that aunt Mabel brings with all the cream cheese and fat, and the string beans with mushroom soup, cream, almonds, and French fried onions. Have plenty of appetizers, like a fresh vegetable tray (or crudités, if you will) with carrots, peppers, celery sticks, and anything else of a vegetable nature you can cut up and chomp.

Low-Fat Stuffing

Serving Size, 1/8 of recipe   Total Servings, 8

Olive oil cooking spray
1 16 oz can fat-free, reduced-sodium chicken broth
1 medium onion, sliced
3 stalks celery, sliced
1 can water chestnuts, sliced
2 cloves garlic, minced
1 medium apple, cubed
1 package stuffing mix

1. Spray the pan with olive oil cooking spray and add a little clear chicken broth.

2. Sauté onions, celery, water chestnuts, garlic, and apple.

3. When all are slightly browned, mix in the stuffing mix and add chicken broth to get the consistency you like.

Exchanges
2 Starch

Calories. 153	**Sodium** . . . . 540 mg
Calories from Fat. 1	**Carbohydrate**. . . . . . . 31 g
Total Fat . . . . 0 g	Dietary Fiber . . . . 4 g
Saturated Fat . . . . 0 g	Sugars . . . . 7 g
Cholesterol . . . . 0 mg	**Protein**. . . . . 4 g

Sweet Potato Casserole

Serving Size, 1/2 cup   Total Servings, 6

3 medium-sized winter squashes
1 Tbsp orange peel
1 tsp cinnamon
1/2 tsp allspice
1 tsp ginger
1/2 tsp cloves
3 Tbsp sugar-free maple syrup
2 Tbsp Smuckers sugar-free apricot preserves
4 packets Equal or Splenda (or to taste)
Butter-flavor cooking spray
3/4 cup Cool Whip Free topping

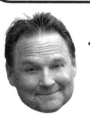

> Set this one out and watch people leave their sugary, marshmallow-topped, butter-ridden, heart-attack-creating dish for your tasty and healthy sweet potato casserole with no potatoes.

1. Start this great tasting sweet potato recipe with absolutely no sweet potatoes. Use some kind of winter squash instead—butternut, acorn, or even pumpkin. Bake until soft. Peel off the cooked skin and put into a food processor or blender.

2. Add orange peel, cinnamon, allspice, ginger, and cloves.

3. Add the maple syrup and apricot preserves. Use Equal or Splenda to sweeten further to taste.

4. Spray a casserole dish with cooking spray, add mixture, and heat in oven. Top with Cool Whip Free topping.

Exchanges
1 Carbohydrate

Calories 67	**Sodium** . . . . 16 mg
Calories from Fat. 7	**Carbohydrate**. . . . . . . 15 g
Total Fat . . . . 1 g	Dietary Fiber . . . . 3 g
Saturated Fat . . . . 0 g	Sugars . . . . 6 g
Cholesterol . . . . 0 mg	**Protein**. . . . . 1 g

Mashed potatoes

Serving Size, 1/6 of recipe   Total Servings, 6

4–6 medium potatoes
2 Tbsp fat-free margarine
3 scallions, chopped
2 oz fat-free cheese, grated
Salt and pepper (*to taste*)
2 garlic cloves, minced
1/2 tsp dill weed

> I love mashed potatoes, but, when I don't want the carbs, I do a variation. I boil cauliflower, put it in the blender, puree it, and season it to taste with fat-free sour cream and chives...but not butter.

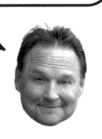

1. Cut and peel potatoes.

2. Boil them to smithereens, then drain.

3. Put drained potatoes in a big bowl and add margarine, scallions, cheese, and salt and pepper. (You can also add garlic if you like garlic mashed potatoes.) Mash entire contents with hand-held masher or use an electric mixer.

4. For presentation, put into casserole dish and garnish with dill weed on top.

Exchanges
1 Starch

Calories. 122		**Sodium** . . . . 104 mg	
Calories from Fat. 1		**Carbohydrate**. . . . . . . 25 g	
Total Fat . . . . 0 g		Dietary Fiber . . . . 2 g	
Saturated Fat . . . . 0 g		Sugars . . . . 3 g	
Cholesterol . . . . 1 mg		**Protein**. . . . . 5 g	

Cranberry relish

Serving Size, 1/20 of recipe   **Total Servings, 20**

1 lb fresh cranberries
1 medium orange
4 packets Equal *(or to taste)*

1. Take the fresh cranberries
   and the whole orange,
   including the peel, and put
   them in the food processor
   on grate. I usually add some
   Equal to it.

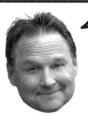

You can't believe how much better this is than that bizarre stuff that comes out of a can.

Exchanges
Free food

Calories 15		**Sodium** . . . . 0 mg	
Calories from Fat. 1		**Carbohydrate** . . . . 4 g	
Total Fat . . . . 0 g		Dietary Fiber . . . . 1 g	
Saturated Fat . . . . 0 g		Sugars . . . . 3 g	
Cholesterol . . . . 0 mg		**Protein** . . . . 0 g	

5-Alarm Chili

Serving Size, 1/6 of recipe   Total Servings, 6

Olive oil in a spray bottle
1 cup onion, chopped
6 cloves garlic, minced
1 lb lean ground turkey or textured soy protein (TSP)
4 8 oz cans no-salt-added tomato sauce
1 20 oz can chopped tomatoes
1 15 oz can pinto beans
1 15 oz can black beans
3 Tbsp chili powder
Hot sauce
Crushed red peppers or cayenne pepper *(or if all else fails, use your wife's pepper spray)*
Italian seasoning spray *(which only works if you're attacked by an Italian)*
3 packages of Equal
Black pepper

1. Brown onions and garlic in a "mist" of olive oil in a nonstick skillet. Add meat and brown.

2. Put tomato sauce and tomatoes and all the beans in a big pot. Add the browned meat mixture.

3. To suit your taste, add any or all of the seasonings, Equal, and black pepper.

4. If you want, you can sauté chopped green pepper and add it. I've also put tofu in. I brown it first in a skillet, and then put it in with the other ingredients.

Exchanges
1-1/2 Starch
2 Lean meat
3 Vegetable

Calories. 304		Sodium . . . . 775 mg	
Calories from Fat. 34		Carbohydrate. . . . . . . 41 g	
Total Fat . . . . 4 g		Dietary Fiber . . . . . . 12 g	
Saturated Fat . . . . 1 g		Sugars . . . . 17 g	
Cholesterol . . . . 49 mg		**Protein**. . . . . 28 g	

Chapter Eight

Between Meal Snacks

When I think back to college, my thoughts turn to the late nights of studying and the late nights of extreme urges for McDonald's cuisine. The employees at the McDonald's on Broad Street in Richmond, Virginia started to know me by name. As my orders for midnight snacks became increasingly larger and larger, I needed to disguise the fact that the massive amounts of food I was ordering were all for me. I had super-sized myself to the limit and still my intense urges for the "golden arches" could not be satisfied.

To soften the painful embarrassment of the clerks rolling their eyes as I ordered enough food for a family of 6, I devised a simple, foolproof plan. I simply used the names of several dorm-mates back at college as the other people whose orders I was picking up. I would take a piece of paper and write several people's names on the list and what they wanted to eat. Little did the guys behind the counter know that I was indeed Paul, Frank, Griff, John, and Nathan all rolled up into this enormous eating machine. There was, however, one fatal flaw to my master plan—I had to order 6 separate drinks in order to protect the intricate undercover operation.

So here I was with all the food I wanted and 6 soda pops. A small price to pay to have a complete and satisfying "Mickey-D" experience. After I changed my lifestyle, my desire for fast food and burgers and fries has unfortunately not changed. You know the McDonald's sign that says how many billions served? It's actually gone down since I've stopped eating there.

Today I use a delicious alternative—as well as some psychological warfare. To create the illusion my stomach seeks, I get a McDonald's burger wrapper and a super-size fries box, wrap up my Fast Food Fantasy (p. 86) and have myself a delicious fast food meal. If I really want to complete the mood, I drive to a McDonald's parking lot and eat it in my car. This may be a bit much, but hey, it works for me!

Nine Out of Ten Experts Agree

In recent years we have learned from the "experts" that things we thought were very healthy for us were suddenly heart attacks in disguise—Chinese food, for example. Who knew that pork deep-fat fried to a golden brown, with bright red artificially colored sweet and sour sauce would be bad for you?

Another report came out that the popcorn in movie theaters is not as healthy as we once thought either. This has nothing to do with the teenager behind the counter who hasn't washed his hands since a cool summer night in '97. It probably had more to do with the type of oil used in the popping, and, of course, that delicious, butter-flavored mystery substance that looks like a cross between butterscotch pudding and orange juice. On top of all that, it was very unhealthy for my wallet to pay as much for a popcorn and drink as I would for a four-person meal at the nearest fast food establishment. I, in my everlasting attempts to fool my body into not feeling it has had to alter anything, have come up with a healthier and much less expensive way to enjoy movie theater popcorn. Check out page 90 for Movie Theater Popcorn that won't make your left arm tingle.

The tricky part, however, is getting into the theater with a non-lethal form of popped corn. Once again, however, I have developed a master plan. First, I put on an overcoat before I buy my ticket. This proves to be very uncomfortable if I'm going to the movies during the summer months or during an unexpected heat wave, but well worth the extra perspiration. Next, I stuff my homemade popcorn in one pocket and a diet soda pop in the other (a cold, well-placed soda pop can be a welcome relief in the aforementioned heat wave). I then proceed to buy my ticket for my favorite film (preferably something that doesn't star anyone from the Survivor cast). I sneak past the pimply-faced ticket taker who undoubtedly wonders what, if anything, is under-neath the overcoat. I take my seat, remove my popcorn and soda, and smile at the fact that it cost me a mere fraction of what it would have cost at the concession stand. It also costs my body a fraction of the fat normally found at the concession stand. Finally—healthy, wealthy, and wise—I sit back and enjoy my munching as I watch the film.

Its Power Enhanced by the Earth's Yellow Sun...

You've probably noticed by now that I use a lot of fat-free cheese. Without a doubt, it's helped me in my impersonation of the incred-ibly shrinking man. However, I must mention that fat-free cheese is a little like kryptonite. It can be a great substitute, but it can also be from outer space and kill Superman. Sometimes it's very difficult to melt fat-free cheese. I kept trying with a particular brand, whose name I cannot remember since I don't buy it any more. It took about 3 hours in the oven to finally get that sucker to melt. I was so excited to look through the oven glass to see the cheese bubbling. I then removed it from the oven to find I had completely disintegrated the other ingredients in my pizza. I suppose there are certain sacrifices you have to be willing to make…

Fast Food Fantasy

Serving Size, 1 Sandwich   Total Servings, 4

1 medium onion, sliced or diced
10 mushrooms, sliced
Nonfat cooking spray
1 lb lean ground turkey
4 slices fat-free cheese
4 hamburger buns
lettuce
1 sliced tomato
pickles
mustard

1. I start by frying up some onions and mushrooms with some Pam cooking spray and a dash of water.

2. I take some very lean ground turkey and make a hamburger filled with the browned mushrooms and onions.

3. Broil the turkey burger and add a slice of fat-free cheese to melt on top. I use a regular hamburger bun and add lettuce and tomato so it can hardly fit in my mouth.

Exchanges
2 Starch
3 Lean meat
1 Vegetable

Calories. 324	**Sodium** . . . . 700 mg	
Calories from Fat. 61	**Carbohydrate**. . . . . . . 32 g	
Total Fat . . . . 7 g	Dietary Fiber . . . . 3 g	
Saturated Fat . . . . 1 g	Sugars . . . . 10 g	
Cholesterol . . . . 62 mg	**Protein**. . . . . 33 g	

French Fries (to complete the Fast Food Fantasy)

Serving Size, 1/4 of recipe   Total Servings, 4

1 potato, cut in narrow strips
Nonfat cooking spray

1. I cut up the potato into narrow strips.

2. Spray a cookie sheet (you got excited over the word cookie, didn't you?) with cooking spray and spread potato strips evenly out on pan.

3. Bake the potatoes till golden brown.

Exchanges
1 Starch

Calories 62		**Sodium** . . . . 4 mg	
Calories from Fat. 1		**Carbohydrate**. . . . . . . 14 g	
Total Fat . . . . 0 g		Dietary Fiber . . . . 1 g	
Saturated Fat . . . . 0 g		Sugars . . . . 1 g	
Cholesterol . . . . 0 mg		**Protein**. . . . . 1 g	

Movie Theater Popcorn

Serving Size, the whole dern thing   **Total Servings, 1**

1/2 cup popcorn kernels *(comes out to about 6 cups when popped)*
A microwave popcorn bowl *(mine is made by Presto)*
Butter flavored cooking spray
Salt substitute *(optional)*

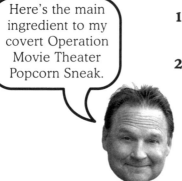

Here's the main ingredient to my covert Operation Movie Theater Popcorn Sneak.

1. Make the popcorn in the microwave with no oil.

2. After it is popped, spray the popcorn with the butter spray and then add salt to your taste. I then put it in a lunch-size brown paper bag and shake it. I also swing the bag over my head, but that's not necessary, I just like to act silly.

Exchanges
2-1/2 Starch

Calories. 184		**Sodium** . . . . 2 mg	
Calories from Fat. 18		**Carbohydrate**. . . . . . . 37 g	
Total Fat . . . . 2 g		Dietary Fiber . . . . 7 g	
Saturated Fat . . . . 0 g		Sugars . . . . 0 g	
Cholesterol . . . . 0 mg		**Protein**. . . . . 6 g	

Frosty Mocha

Serving Size, 1/4 recipe   **Total Servings, 4**

1/2 cup no-sugar-added, reduced-fat vanilla ice cream
1 package Swiss Miss Diet Cocoa
1 cup fat-free half-and-half
2 cups of coffee
1/2 tsp cinnamon
4–6 ice cubes

1. Put all the ingredients into a blender and blend to a sweet mocha shade.

2. I love iced mochas and I especially love the Starbuck's original. To complete this recipe, I try to finagle a Starbuck's cup and pour the finished product in to that. It's healthier, and I save approximately $4,376 a week.*

Exchanges
1 Carbohydrate

Calories 86	**Sodium** . . . . 101 mg	
Calories from Fat. 20	**Carbohydrate**. . . . . . . 13 g	
Total Fat . . . . 2 g	Dietary Fiber . . . . 0 g	
Saturated Fat . . . . 1 g	Sugars . . . . 5 g	
Cholesterol . . . . 10 mg	**Protein**. . . . . 3 g	

---

* I have an excellent relationship with my local Starbuck's, which I visit every day for coffee and a baguette. And I pay for them!

Peanut Butter and Jelly Sandwich

Serving Size, 1 Sandwich   Total Servings, 1

2 slices of bread
2 Tbsp "altered" peanut butter *(see below)*
2 Tbsp sugar-free Smuckers apricot jam

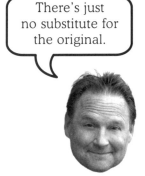

There's just no substitute for the original.

1. Do you really need directions? Okay, I will give you this inside tip—I buy natural peanut butter and pour the oil off. I label it "altered peanut butter" and marvel at the density. It can double as an anchor for a fishing vessel. You're going to need plenty of liquid to get that down. And I like Smuckers sugar-free jam, too. The apricot is best.

Exchanges
1 Carbohydrate
2 Starch
1 High fat meat
1/2 Fat

Calories. 338	**Sodium** . . . . 476 mg
Calories from Fat. . . . 121	**Carbohydrate**. . . . . . . 45 g
Total Fat. . . . . 13 g	Dietary Fiber . . . . 6 g
Saturated Fat . . . . 2 g	Sugars . . . . 7 g
Cholesterol . . . . 0 mg	**Protein**. . . . . 13 g

Quick Pizza

Serving Size, 1/2 of recipe   Total Servings, 2

1 whole-wheat pita bread
1/2 cup spaghetti sauce
1 cup mixed chopped veggies
1/2 cup low-fat cheese, grated

1. Cover pita with spaghetti sauce.
   Sprinkle veggies on top.
   Sprinkle cheese over all.

2. Bake it at 400° F for 10 minutes.
   Broil it for 2 or 3 minutes, or
   until the cheese melts and
   makes everything toasty.

For the feel of take-out pizza, I hire somebody to bring this to my door. But I always get it free because I pretend they didn't get there in 30 minutes.

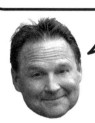

Exchanges
1 Starch
3 Vegetable
2 Fat

Calories. 238	**Sodium** . . . . 619 mg
Calories from Fat. 89	**Carbohydrate**. . . . . . . 30 g
Total Fat. . . . . 10 g	Dietary Fiber . . . . 5 g
Saturated Fat . . . . 4 g	Sugars . . . . 5 g
Cholesterol . . . . 20 mg	**Protein**. . . . . 12 g

Chapter Nine

Soups and Salads

I have lots of soups. Soup is a great way to get lots of vegetables that you wouldn't eat otherwise. When I started making soups, I got into more exotic stuff and left macaroni and cheese and fast food stuff behind. I started using spices I'd never even heard of, just for flavors in the soups. I would make a Mexican soup and an Indian soup, a chicken curry vegetable noodle soup—oh my gosh, it was to die for. There are actually an infinite number of soup recipes in the world and I never make the same one twice.

Chicken Curry Vegetable Noodle Soup

Serving Size, 1/4 of recipe   **Total Servings, 4**

1 quart water
3 uncooked boneless, skinless chicken breasts
2 cups any vegetables you like, chopped or sliced
1/2 cup noodles or pasta
1/2 to 1 tsp curry powder or garam masala
1/2 tsp ground cardamom
Salt and pepper (*to taste*)
3 packets Equal
1 Tbsp lemon juice (*for the sweet and sour pungent flavor*)

You can make Lemon grass soup with this recipe by adding 1/2 cup coconut milk. It has a great flavor, but even though it's a vegetable fat, it is a saturated fat.

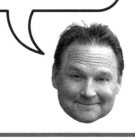

1. Put water in a large pot to boil. Chop chicken into bite sized pieces and add to the pot.

2. Chop vegetables, such as green peppers, red peppers, onions, mushrooms, spinach, zucchini, and add to the soup pot. Simmer for 25 minutes.

3. Add noodles, spices, and Equal. Let simmer for 10 more minutes or until noodles are soft.

Exchanges
1/2 Carbohydrates
3 Very lean meat

Calories. 137	**Sodium** . . . . 65 mg
Calories from Fat. 14	**Carbohydrate**. . . . . 9 g
Total Fat . . . . 2 g	Dietary Fiber . . . . 2 g
Saturated Fat . . . . 0 g	Sugars . . . . 4 g
Cholesterol . . . . 52 mg	**Protein**. . . . . 21 g

Sweet and Sour Soup

Serving Size, 1/8 of recipe   **Total Servings, 8**

3 uncooked boneless, skinless chicken breasts
3 cups of any kind of vegetables you like
1 46 oz can V-8 juice
46 oz water *(V-8 and water are mixed 1 to 1)*
1 Tbsp fresh lemon juice
4 packets Equal

1. Mix all ingredients together in a big pot, and bring them to a boil. Simmer for 30 to 45 minutes. Season to suit your taste.

Exchanges
1 Very lean meat
2 Vegetable

Calories 94		**Sodium** . . . . 445 mg	
Calories from Fat. 7		**Carbohydrate**. . . . . . . 11 g	
Total Fat . . . . 1 g		Dietary Fiber . . . . 1 g	
Saturated Fat . . . . 0 g		Sugars . . . . 7 g	
Cholesterol . . . . 24 mg		**Protein**. . . . . 11 g	

Another Good Soup

Serving Size, 1/4 of recipe   **Total Servings, 4**

1 large acorn squash
1 16 oz can fat-free, reduced-sodium chicken broth
1/2 cup fat-free half-and-half
1-1/2-inch piece ginger, grated
1/4 tsp grated nutmeg
Salt and pepper (*to taste*)
Dash of dill or peppermint (*optional*)

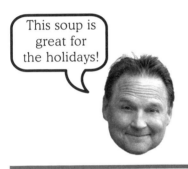

This soup is great for the holidays!

1. Cook the acorn squash and puree it. Add chicken broth and fat-free half-and-half. Stir over low heat, do not boil.

2. Add ginger and nutmeg, salt and pepper, garnish with dill or peppermint.

Exchanges
1 Starch

Calories 93	**Sodium** . . . . 299 mg
Calories from Fat. 13	**Carbohydrate** . . . . 18 g
Total Fat . . . . 1 g	Dietary Fiber . . . . 5 g
Saturated Fat . . . . 0 g	Sugars . . . . 7 g
Cholesterol . . . . 2 mg	**Protein**. . . . . 3 g

Waldorf Salad

Serving Size, 1/8 of recipe   Total Servings, 8

1 large package sugar-free lime Jell-O *(or 2 regular packages)*
1 6 oz can water chestnuts, chopped *(they're crunchy but have no fat, so they replace the walnuts)*
1 medium apple, chopped
1/2 cup nonfat yogurt

1. Make Jell-O according to package directions. Refrigerate for 30 minutes until slightly thickened.

2. Add the rest of the ingredients, and mix well. Refrigerate until firm.

This makes a portion for 8 people—and I would eat the whole thing. But the whole thing only has about 300 calories. It really fills you up, too.

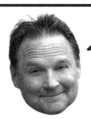

Exchanges
1/2 Carbohydrate

Calories 39	**Sodium** . . . . 71 mg
Calories from Fat. 1	**Carbohydrate**. . . . . 8 g
Total Fat . . . . 0 g	Dietary Fiber . . . . 1 g
Saturated Fat . . . . 0 g	Sugars . . . . 5 g
Cholesterol . . . . 0 mg	**Protein**. . . . . 2 g

My High Falutin' Salad

Serving Size, 1/8 of recipe   Total Servings, 8

1 large bunch of field greens *(baby spring field greens, raddichio, arugula, endive, etc.)*
1 pint grape tomatoes
2 medium yellow bell peppers
6 green onions or scallions
1 medium pear
1/2 cup walnuts
4 oz feta cheese
1/4 cup balsamic vinaigrette dressing

1. Wash the greens, spin dry, and tear into bite-sized pieces.

2. Cut up the vegetables and pear. Chop the walnuts, crumble the feta cheese.

3. Toss everything together. Sprinkle dressing over the salad lightly (finding a lower fat vinaigrette will lower the calories quite a bit).

Exchanges
1/2 Carbohydrate
1 Vegetable
2 Fat

Calories. 145		**Sodium** . . . . 243 mg	
Calories from Fat. 87		**Carbohydrate**. . . . . . . 12 g	
Total Fat. . . . . 10 g		Dietary Fiber . . . . 3 g	
Saturated Fat . . . . 2 g		Sugars . . . . 7 g	
Cholesterol . . . . . . 12 mg		**Protein**. . . . . 4 g	

Chapter Ten

What It's Like Being Thin

There are certain indignities you have to endure when you're a fat person. One of the worst—besides being asked to get off an amusement park ride—is flying on an airplane. The look on peoples' faces when they see you coming toward them down the aisle is astonishing. It's as if they think you may grab their peanut snacks when they're not looking (well, once the guy went to the bathroom and I just had a craving for those honey roasted wonders...). But for the most part, if you keep your hands and feet away from our mouths, you're perfectly safe.

Another fear that "slim" folk have is the fear that we'll be sitting next to them. I do understand the laws of physics and the idea of "encroaching on someone else's seat." I also understand the laws of physics when it comes to buckling up the seat belts. It just ain't gonna happen with a pleasantly plump, 320-pound guy like I was. I had to have the Seat Belt Extension—which is like putting two seat belts together—amazingly, it's something they never show on the little films of the smiling customers explaining how to hook up.

One of the funnier things I ever encountered was when I ordered a seat belt extension over the phone for a trip to New York City I had to take in the mid 1980s. The attendant on the other end of the line made all the arrangements for me, and then asked if I would be needing an extension for the return trip 7 days later. At that point, I demanded she tell me about this amazing diet she knew where I could magically lose 100 pounds in 7 days. I'd be more than happy to take everything I owned and invest it in this miracle diet.

On another occasion I boarded a plane and found myself sitting with a convention of Herbalife salesman. They all had buttons on saying, "Ask me how to lose weight." They saw me coming from a mile away, literally. When I got off the plane, I had purchased about $500 worth of Herbalife products. By the way...it didn't work for me!

A lot of slimmer people can't even fathom why fat people can't eat a normal portion size, or why people eat when they're lonely, depressed, happy, anxious, bored, or celebrating Lincoln's mother's birthday. I understand their feelings. Just as they can't understand my addiction, I can't understand the craving for alcohol, or the fear of flying, or the need to inhale a cloud of poison smoke into your lungs. So, I do understand the disgust and the misunderstanding about people like me, people who'd eat something they didn't even like just to have that feeling of satisfaction and security. The battle of the bulge is something I know very well. Actually, it's not a battle for me—it's a war!

It's funny that even after six years of being thin, there is still a fat person inside me trying to get out. I look at myself in the mirror, and I don't even recognize the person standing there. I see myself as wearing a "thin person" disguise. My mind still thinks as a fat person. I pick restaurants where I know I'll be able to get enough food—albeit, healthy food—to eat. If I feel my pants are too tight, I start to get paranoid that I'm gaining weight even though the scale says I'm still between 175 and 180.

I was doing the television series *Babylon 5* when I decided to lose weight. I started dropping pounds toward the end of one season, and then there was a four-month hiatus. I never mentioned to anyone that I was on a diet. I showed up on the first day of work for the new season, and my alien costume was in my dressing room as always. I put on the costume, and it was hanging off of me! I called the wardrobe people in and asked if there was something they could do about this. They almost died when they saw that the costume was roomy enough to fit a couple more actors inside along with me. They furiously pinned me from the back to take in the costume as much as they could. If you watch the first episode of season four, my character never turns his back to the camera. After that show, they took the costume in, and I was able

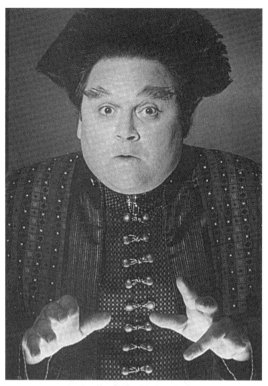

Babylon 5, Before and After

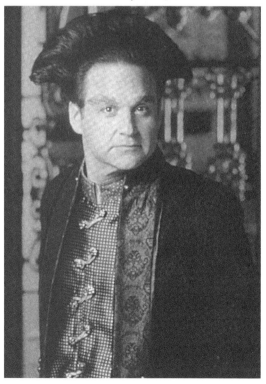

to walk past the camera again. After the show, they said to me, "Don't ever do that to us again." I promised I would not be losing an additional 100 pounds.

In the cast photo of *Babylon 5* for season four, I couldn't find myself when the pictures came out. I was quite upset because I thought they had fired me, decided not to tell me, and just airbrushed me out of the picture. But I was in the picture—I just didn't recognize myself.

Sweating

I also noticed that I stopped sweating profusely once I got thin. I used to sweat all the time. I remember getting a job in a commercial for a new product for Frito Lay. It was being filmed in July in Los Angeles. It happened to be a rather unseasonably cool day for July, and I overheard the ad executive say to the director, "See, we lucked out with the weather. You thought he was going to sweat like a pig!" It's weird because I was concerned for the guy's feelings. I was worried that he was going to get upset if he knew that I had overheard them.

The bad thing about getting too hot and sweaty when you're overweight is that it doesn't fit with the usual fashion choices of fat people. The idea is to cover up as much as possible when you're fat, but the extra layers of clothing add extra heat. Sure, I would have liked to go outside wearing shorts, *sans* shirt, but I don't think the rest of the world would want that (nor would I want the ridicule).

I remember well the two hottest times I ever had to endure. Once was when I was doing a film in Dallas in August. It was a Columbia Pictures film called *Silent Rage* starring Chuck Norris and me. It was somewhere around 116° in the shade. Mix that with a 320-pound guy, and you've got yourself one hot cowboy. I thought I was going to die, or I had already died, and this was

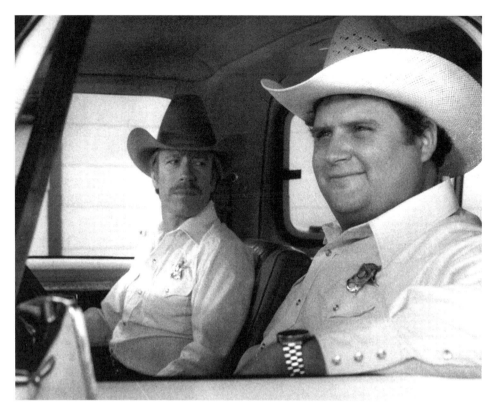

Broiling in my own broth on the set of *Silent Rage*, with Chuck Norris.
(Picture courtesy of Columbia Pictures.)

Hell. All the local folks kept telling me the same thing, "Well, at least you're not in Houston."

I experienced another heat wave when I was doing an episode of *St. Elsewhere*. Even though the series took place in Boston, the show was actually shot in Los Angeles. One July afternoon, I had to do a scene where my character's car was caught in a snow bank. Now, you're asking, how do you get a car stuck in the snow in Los Angeles in July? In Hollywood, anything is possible. They had a truck with equipment that would make snow and then blow it all over the car. They built up a snow bank where I was supposed to be stuck. My costume was a heavy overcoat, hat, gloves, and scarf. So, I had to dig my car out of the snow on a supposedly bitter cold day in Boston, when really it was sweltering hot with the temperature in the upper 90s in Los Angeles. I think I lost 10 pounds that day just from all the sweat. But never fear; there was a restaurant across the street from the studio that was famous for their roast pork and plum sauce sandwich on garlic bread. I had no problem replenishing the 10 pounds.

Behind the Scenes

The actor Wayne Knight ("Newman" on *Seinfeld*), sent me a note one time through a mutual acquaintance that said, "Stop getting my parts." I guess people thought I looked like him. I had so many people tell me they thought I was funny on Seinfeld. Now we look nothing alike. I worked with him on *Buzz Lightyear* after I lost weight. He plays the bad guy, and of course, I am the fat, but naïve and lovable alien.

You might think the most dangerous part of movie making is the terrific stunts. But the real danger for me was something called the craft service table. That's the snack table set up for the cast and crew, so there is always something to eat on the set. Bagels and doughnuts in the morning, and an endless supply of snacks the rest of the day. It was deadly for me to even walk by the craft service table. The food would just call to me; lying there open, naked, and just for the taking. The M&Ms would scream out my name like paparazzi. Especially the green ones. I would defiantly walk by, but at the end of the day (because I was a notorious closet eater), I would throw some snacks in my brief-case when no one was around and eat them on the way home.

As I mentioned before, I tried to use psychological tricks when I started my diet. I would bring healthy snacks from home and place them on the table. I would place them as far away from the peanut butter cookies as possible (I am like putty when it comes to peanut butter cookies). I even started baking my diet lemon poppy seed muffin loaf (p. 53) and bringing it to the set.

I put a sign on the loaf that read, "This is sugar free and fat free." Someone added one more line when I wasn't looking—"Taste free, too." People laughed and joked about it, but little by little, they started to taste the lemon poppy seed cake, and it became very popular. I started to sell them for $3 a loaf, which supplemented my acting income.

I worked with a producer recently who had the forethought to send out fact sheets for the cast and crew on what they liked for snacks. When enough people requested healthier snacks, they showed up on the craft service table.

I still have to remind myself of the inherent dangers in "sugar free" or "fat free" or "eat as much as you like." If I see that kind of label, or even if the product has "healthy" in the name, it's all over for me. Don't put a box of Snackwell cookies in front of me. I think I'm snacking healthy AND well—and I eat them all, which is not a true serving size. Or how about "no-sugar-added" ice cream? I used to eat the entire quart. A pregnant woman might overeat and say, "I'm eating for two." But when I overate, I'd say, "I'm eating for an entire litter." With diabetes, you have to watch fat-free products, because they have even more carbohydrate in them than the regular version of the food. That will send your blood sugar soaring.

Dinner Parties, Get-Togethers, and Other Gutbusters

Once I became thin, I had problems with giving dinner parties. I couldn't make everyone follow my lifestyle choices. I'd do baked brie with raspberries and almonds on top (a beloved "company" appetizer), but I'd also have the salsa and baked chips and vegetable crudities. I'd make onion dip with the soup mix, but I'd use nonfat sour cream. For dessert, I'd make them strawberry shortcake, and I'd have diet shortcake with sugar-free pound cake, Cool Whip Free, and fresh strawberries. I'd pass around their servings, and then bring out mine. They'd say, "Yours looks different from ours." My serving was bigger than theirs was, and they thought I was being a very ungracious host! Bigger is always better, especially when it comes to dessert.

I was pretty relentless when I was trying to lose weight. I remember once being invited to a ranch theme party where they served BBQ beans and ribs and mayo-laden coleslaw and steak fries. There was absolutely nothing I could eat. How was I going to make it through this dinner and party for 6 hours with nothing to eat?! Then I saw the oasis in the vast desert of fat-dripping BBQ ribs. As I said, the theme of the party was southwestern, and the centerpieces on the tables were multi-colored peppers. Red

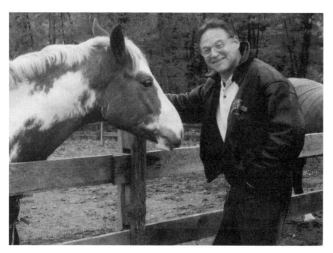

peppers, yellow peppers, green peppers. So I did what I had to do. I ate every centerpiece. I was already known in my community as the guy in showbiz, but after I ate the centerpieces, I was the talk of the town.

Eating healthy is possible everywhere... whether you're at home or "home on the range!"

In the Spirit

To take yourself by the scruff of the neck and completely change your life requires hope, and there's got to be a spiritual aspect to that. You are more than just that poor tired body. I didn't look towards a Supreme Being "out there" to help me. I have a Supreme Being who is part of me. And I look for the ultimate good person deep inside me—the one who does everything right.

(Admittedly, he doesn't always come out.) That's my new religion—to be the kindest, nicest person I possibly can and to help others. To touch as many people's lives as I can. And I look toward that Supreme Being. Some people might say, "Wow, he's the most conceited person I've ever met." But it's inside me. I don't look outside myself for spiritual guidance, I look inside; it's the only place to know you're connected. Whenever you think the power source is "out there," you're always weak.

Taking control of my life has made me a better person in little ways, like being really honest—with myself and others. I think you can't really start to lose weight until you get honest with yourself. I wasn't always so honest before. I never did anything illegal, but if I was given too much change at a store, I'd think, "Hey, I just got $5." Now, I'd return it immediately. It's just being considerate of my fellow human beings.

About 7 years ago, I went back to school and studied psychology, just for personal growth (mentally, not expanding at the waistline). While I was doing that, I decided I wanted another challenge in my life and a way to use my new found skills as a student therapist, so I started teaching at Juvenile Hall. I worked there for about a year and a half until I got the role on *Babylon 5* and had to stop teaching. I had a great time teaching because I felt I was reaching some of the students. About 86% of the kids there would end up back in jail, but I still found it rewarding trying to get to the 14% who wanted to change their lives.

Recently I have gone back to teaching occasionally. I wish I had more time to do it, but I teach when I have a day here and there. The kids don't recognize me, but they are familiar with my voice because of all the cartoons that I do. I tell them the films that I was in and then show them the picture I always carry around with me. It's a picture of me in the movie *Midnight Madness* that I did with Michael J. Fox. This was a film I did when

I was 320 pounds. It's a rough photo with a terribly unflattering pose showing several chins hanging from my face. The kids refuse to believe that it is me. They think that it was some Hollywood magic special effects make-up job, like Eddie Murphy's in *The Nutty Professor*. The kids always end up persuading me to do cartoon voices for them. But it doesn't really look good when the administrator of the prison walks in on your class and you're doing voices from *The Little Mermaid* for the inmates.

Up in the Air

When ordering meals on airlines, I never order a diabetic meal. I have no idea where they got their nutrition training but I'm pretty sure it may have been the Diabetic Coma Institute! I once got a regular yogurt with a huge plate of fruit, orange juice, a bagel with cream cheese, and cereal. All carbs. They did give me Sweet 'N Low instead of sugar, so I guess that's where the diabetic part of the meal came in. Now I always order the low-fat meal, and it's usually pretty good for diabetes, too.

Before I was on my diet, I used to call up and order a special meal of just junk food. They laughed and thought I was kidding. I wasn't. And you know how they always say people with diabetes should bring enough food to have on their flight just in case you can't eat the food they serve or they forget your special meal? Well, I kind of overdid it in case the flight was cancelled, and there was no food around for miles. I packed an entire suitcase with a meal for a family of eight with built-in seconds. I was usually charged for excess luggage.

Even with all the food I packed and the extra charges, I still got off cheaper than buying a bagel and a cup of coffee at airport prices. I once had to make payments on a cheeseburger and fries. I would have ordered a drink with it, but I didn't think I could qualify for the larger loan.

Captain Kirk, We've Got Klingons

Needless to say, science fiction fans are also big fans of the internet and all the fan-based sites for their favorite shows. You can always tell a sci-fi fan because they know more about your life than you do. I once had a guy come up to me and start doing imperson-ations. He said, "Guess who I'm doing." After several failed attempts at trying to guess who he was impersonating, I finally swallowed my pride and gave up. He shouted out with much enthusiasm, "I'm doing YOU!" I was so embarrassed.

On the internet fan site, there were all these rumors circulating after I had lost weight that I was dying of cancer and that's why I looked so thin. I went on the chat room to convince all the fans that I

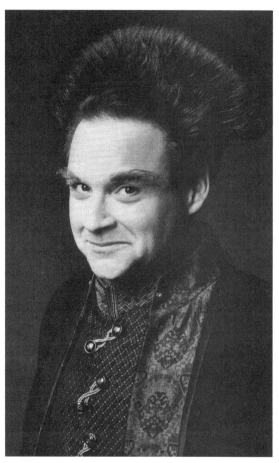

I'm just your everyday healthy alien, no "space sickness" here! (*Babylon 5*)

was alive and well and had just gone on a diet. I was not dying of some strange outer space cancer that I had contracted on the ship. (They really believe I lived on a spaceship.)

I used to do sci-fi conventions, and fans would come up to my autograph table and ask me, "Do you know when Stephen Furst will be returning to sign autographs?"

I would jokingly say, "Sooner than you think."

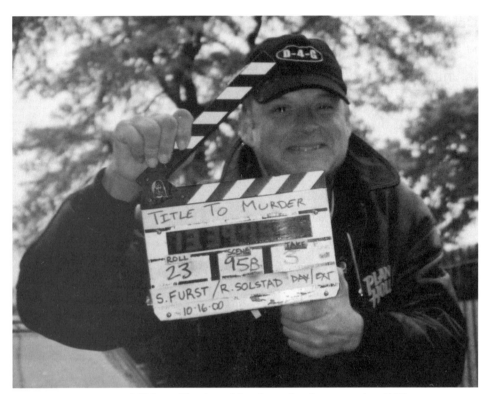

Directing on the set of *Title to Murder* while shamelessly promoting D4G.

Flab or Fame?

People always ask if losing weight has hurt my acting career. I honestly have to say that I think it did. I had already started moving into directing when I decided to lose weight, but I'm sure losing weight had an effect. I am now more nonspecific as a character. I just auditioned for a role recently, and I felt that I had done well. But I noticed in the waiting room that there were all sorts of actors of all different sizes and shapes and colors. I did well, but they went with a different color.

That still doesn't beat the time I landed my very first acting job for a commercial for Marx Toys company. I called all my family back in Virginia to tell them I was on my way to becoming a huge star. I spent an entire week's salary as a pizza delivery guy calling everybody I knew. The next day my agent called me and said, "Are you sitting down? I have some bad news."

What could it be? I had just gotten a national commercial; I already had big plans for all the money I was about to make.

"They replaced you."

"What do you mean 'they replaced me?' I was the best guy for the role." My agent then told me the horrifying news.

"They went a different way. They decided to use a chimpanzee."

Like any other actor would have, I replied, "I can do chimpanzee better than anybody!"

I also think that age has a lot to do with the acting roles not being as plentiful. This is very much a youth-oriented business. When the youth starts to fade, so do some of the better roles. You have older actors who are Academy Award winners, like Richard Dreyfuss and Sally Fields, doing television. When stars like that do a TV series, there is a trickle-down effect. The next level of actors, such as myself who used to be in a TV series, are now relegated to the supporting and guest star roles. That's what they call "Showbiz."

Chapter Eleven

Eating Out Tips

Even though I'm thin now, you can always tell the fat person inside still lives on. When I go out to dinner with friends, they inevitably leave part of their meal on the plate. I may eat a healthy selection, but I never leave anything on my plate. (I think it goes back to all those starving children overseas that my parents told me about. I always wondered how stuffing my face helped those starving kids, but who was I to question my parents?) So, after the meal, the waiter typically asks if they want a doggie-bag, and they have the audacity to say "no." Didn't they know what wonderful hour would come later when no one was looking? Didn't they realize what a snack that would make? Immediately, I request a doggie-bag for their leftovers, and ask the waiter to see if the next table over is going to leave part of their meal, too.

One of my favorite restaurants is Wood Ranch BBQ in my hometown. Every Monday night, for *Monday Night Football,* they would have an all-you-can-eat beef rib night. And the ribs came with little french fried onions and peanut coleslaw and rolls drenched in garlic butter. I would get there for the pre-game show and stay till the post-game interviews were complete. I even wrote to the NFL once to ask if they could extend the season. It was always a sad day when the regular season ended, and I knew I was going to have to wait another 8 months for a Monday night kickoff.

✳ ✳ ✳

Even after my dad died of a heart attack (brought on by his diabetes), my mother and I went to New York City for a vacation and ate our way from one end of Times Square to the other. There was Lindy's world famous cheesecake. I just had to find out for myself how this cheesecake became so famous. After one bite, I realized that I had just eaten the Barbara Streisand of cheesecakes. Then there was Mama Leone's Italian restaurant, where they brought you a loaf of cheese and great bread before

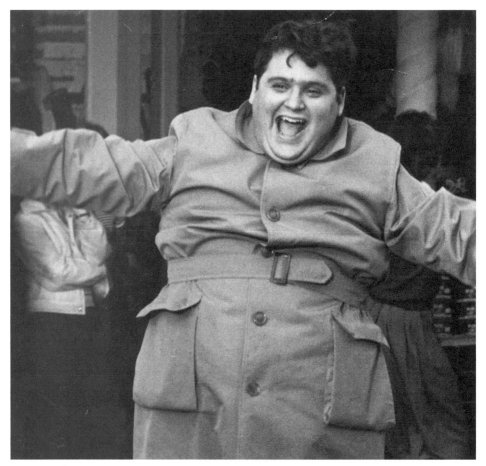

Jumping for joy as "Flounder" in *Animal House*...or was it the cheesecake?

the meal. They're closed now, but it had nothing to do with me and all that missing cheese, I promise. And then, of course, there were Nathan's Hot Dogs. I was so moved by that experience I named my first son Nathan. Of course, between eating establishments, there were food street vendors to quell any hunger pains that might have developed in transit from one location to the next. The pretzels, chestnuts, and potato knishes. Finally, a city after my own heart…literally!

Even though my favorite restaurants back then, and even now, are the all-you-can-eat places, I try to steer clear of any place with a buffet. It's like telling an alcoholic to go into a bar and order an iced tea. One time I was actually asked to leave a buffet. I was merely inquiring when the lunch buffet stopped and when they were going to bring out the dinner selections. Of course, I had already eaten lunch there and was trying to stall till the dinner platters were on their way. They were onto me.

Eating out at a restaurant doesn't have to be hard. Just tell them what you want and don't try to fool yourself. People tell me that they ate healthy today. I ask what they ordered. "I only had a salad for lunch," they say. Come to find out, it was a Cobb salad, or a Chef salad with cups of blue cheese dressing. When I go to a restaurant, I ask for a chef salad with no bacon, ham or cheese. I ask for extra turkey and extra veggies. I make my own dressing at the table with olive oil, balsamic vinegar, and Dijon mustard. I add one packet of Equal. People say to me, "You put equal on your salad?" I tell them to look at the ingredients on their salad dressing bottle and see how much sugar is in it.

I hardly ever order straight off the menu. I always ask for "no butter" or "no oil" or "Could you put that on the side, please?" or "Can I have salsa on my baked potato instead of butter, sour cream, and bacon bits?" I also drink big glasses of iced tea. But be careful with the iced tea. If you're in the South or Canada, they sweeten the iced tea with pounds of sugar and you're liable to get something closer to hummingbird food than actual tea.

Sometimes my boys ask me, "For once, would it kill you to just order off the menu?"

I say, "As a matter of fact, it will." After all, I am the same guy who sent back a salad with thousand island dressing on it because I told the waitress I could only count 879 islands. I have no idea why I embarrass my kids.

How to Eat Out—A Guide for Each Cuisine

Mexican

For me, eating low fat Mexican food is the greatest challenge of all. Fajitas are good because they're vegetables and meat. I always ask if there's lard in the tortillas. If there's lard in them, I might as well just skip the process of eating them and cram them directly into my arteries.

Japanese

Ah, sushi. It is my absolute, all-time favorite food. If you don't like raw fish, try the California roll and vegetable rolls. Stay away from Tempura and Teriyaki—they can really mess with your fat grams for the day.

Chinese

Watch out for the gargantuan amounts of oil they use. I get steamed, white meat chicken with steamed vegetables and steamed rice. I ask that they not use oil when preparing any of it. I use soy sauce and pepper and the Chinese chili sauce to make it spicy. And in this particular case, I don't use Equal.

Italian

I can have pasta, but I stay away from red meats like veal and beef and sausage. I'll have pasta with tomatoes and olive oil, but I don't use cheese. I put chili peppers on it, too. And I have a big salad. I love salad bars. I go for all the lower-fat stuff. I get to chew a lot, it fills me up, and the calories are low.

The Tao of Restaurant Eating

Basically, no matter where you eat, it boils down to choices. Am I going to go for the fatty muffins, or for a piece of sourdough bread? Am I going to get Kung Pao Chicken fried in sesame oil with peanuts, or something steamed with lots of vegetables? I can go to McDonald's now and get a char-broiled chicken sandwich with no condiments. The dangerous time has passed. I can make the right choices without even thinking about it. I have changed my whole lifestyle. I've even gotten into feng shui—I rearrange my carbohydrates to face East.

When ordering in a restaurant, I never get embarrassed. Whenever I ask for something special, I just say that I'll pay for it. Please throw in three portions of broccoli—I'll pay for it. Like recently, we ate out at Old Ebbitt Grill in Washington, D.C., and my grilled chicken sandwich came with French fries. I said, "Is there anything you can do instead of French fries?" (I love it when people say, "Well, we can give you mashed potatoes and gravy." That's not helping.) So he said, "We can give you fresh fruit." Great! I had the chicken sandwich and the fruit, and I was full. I ate the garnishes, too!

You see, I've realized that the look I get from the waiter when I order extra vegetables is better than the look I got from the McDonald's crew when I'd order enough food for an entire football team. I'd rather be embarrassed by ordering three extra portions of broccoli than suffer the humiliation I once went through when ordering fast-food with my 10-year-old son. We were at a drive-in and I ordered 6 tacos because they were on special. My son yelled out, "You're going to eat 6 tacos?!" I thought quickly on my feet, and used the line about starving children overseas…

Oh, the Places You'll Go…

I feel like my life has been a wonderful journey so far. I have been able to make a living doing something I adore doing. I have traveled to places that I thought I would never go. I have met people that I thought I would only see in fantasies. What other guy has been in college with a poster of Bette Midler over his bed, and one year later been taken out to dinner by Bette at a Japanese restaurant in New York City?

I have rescued myself from slow suicide, as the doctor put it, and been able to watch my children grow up and even get married. I'm not a believer in miracles so much as a believer in fate. I feel that I hit bottom when I did because of fate, so that I can bring what I've been through to help other people in similar situations. I have been through those days when things seem so dark and finally you say, "I can't stand being sick all the time." That's the day you wake up and say, "I'm going to take control of my diabetes, rather than let my diabetes take control of me."

Chapter Twelve

Sports? Exercise?

I just got a dog, and he's already been wonderful for raising my exercise level. I'm outside and walking so much more just because of him. Oh, by the way, he's a chocolate lab—a sugar-free chocolate lab. His name is Starbuck. I got him at the pound, and when I saw his name, I knew we were destined for each other. It was kismet.

Because I used to be a closet eater (and amazingly adept at lying to myself), I could use that lame excuse of having an overactive thyroid for my weight problem. That story stuck with me

for years like peanut butter on the roof of your mouth, until a doctor told me I definitely didn't have a thyroid problem. I said, "Are you kiddin'? I don't have a thyroid problem? Give it to me straight, doc. What do I have?"

His answer was simple, yet so complex. "You eat too much."

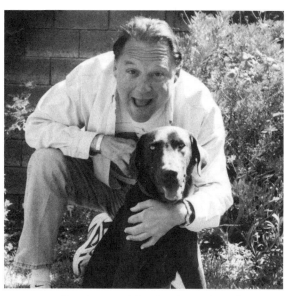

Stephen and Starbuck, workout buddies.

I was stunned. Immediately I asked, "Is there a cure or some medicine I can take?" I was looking for an easy answer. I wanted to take a magic pill and drop 50 pounds by the following Tuesday. I wanted to hook myself up to a mini-electrocution machine and have a six pack stomach overnight. I actually tried that. I was promised, for $59.99 plus shipping and handling, that this tiny little electric machine would send my stomach muscles into convulsions, and I would be able to change my look from the six-tire Michelin Man to a lean model fit for the cover of *Men's Health* magazine.

I quickly found out there was no miracle pill. And no little machine to give me a ripped stomach of muscles. I had to diet, and even worse, I actually had to, gulp, exercise. Exercise is a word I have trouble even saying. I even had a hard time typing it for this book. Exercise to me is right up there with things like the no-return policy, or buying insurance, or "some assembly required," or my favorite, "but, Dad, all the kids are doing it." However, it's a fact of life, no matter how awful it sounds. I remember saying on a movie set one time to fellow actor, Tim Matheson, "I can't understand why I'm fat, because I really don't eat that much." I left out the part about eating when no one was looking.

He told me it was simple, "If you take in more calories than you burn, you'll gain weight."

Wait a second! That was just too simple an answer. Didn't he know he was dealing with a professional and covert overeater here?

Just as I had a solution for dieting and fooling myself into thinking I was still eating what I wanted, I devised ways to do things I felt were fun until I got the strength up to actually exercise. (I mean, the best money I had ever spent for a household item was for a stationary bike. Do you know how much clothes a stationary bike can hold?) I started walking the dog. But I didn't have a dog, so that was my first problem. I would borrow the neighbor's dog, a Chinese Sharpei named Ripples. I identified with the dog because it's exactly what I looked like before I lost weight. I would walk it, or sometimes it would briskly walk me.

As I started getting in better shape, I would bicycle down to Starbuck's. I was motivated to take the bike ride because of the reward at the other end. I think this is technically referred to as "Pavlov's latte."

When I finally got up enough nerve to go to the gym, I had to swallow my pride and work out next to women who could bench press me. Meanwhile, I slyly slipped the 5-pound weight on the bicep curl machine. But I kept at it and have worked up to a much better level of mediocrity. There's one problem with my gym, however—it happens to be next door to a gourmet market. For the first six months, I thought I was schizophrenic—I swore I heard the pastries calling me through the wall.

One thing that helps is having a friend to work out with, or accompany you for a walk. After you finish gossiping, the exercise is over and you realize you hardly felt a thing. My feet are sensitive to infection, like most people with diabetes. When I walked on the treadmill my shoes rubbed against my feet too much, so I switched to using the stairmaster or a stationary bike. I strap on my favorite music, put a wad of sugar-free gum in my mouth, and I go for it. For people with severe neuropathy, you can wear water shoes and walk laps in a pool for exercise.

Hopping on the stairmaster is a lot different from the exercise I used to get, which was pretty much limited to walking from the couch to the refrigerator during a commercial break. If I had for-gotten something and had to go back to the fridge, that counted as my exercise for the next day. I also found out that you burn

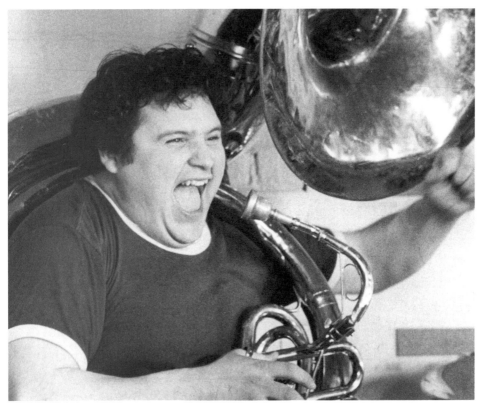

If only I had known how exciting it can be to lose weight! (*Take Down*, Disney)

approximately one calorie using the remote. With all the channels today, think of all the calories I could have burned. I get exhausted just thinking about it.

Even after working out for years, there's still something I've yet to work up the courage to do—shower with the other guys at the gym. Some habits die hard. God, how I dreaded my 7th grade gym teacher when he made everyone shower after gym class. I'm sure he is in heaven now making sure everyone has a shower before they enter the pearly gates.

Before I went to the gym, I was so motivated to start exercising, but I just couldn't get up enough energy. I even hired some neighborhood bullies to chase me. But even that didn't work. I gave up, gave them my lunch money, went back home, and made a sandwich to drown my sorrows at not being successful.

You Can Make a Game Out of It

If you still find the gym too daunting, remember you don't have to go to the gym to have a workout. Household chores count, too. Take mowing the lawn for example, but not on one of those Cadillac riding lawnmowers. For a real workout, try a stand-up push-mower. You know, the ones that take forever to start.

For me, I tried to make working out fun because that way I didn't notice the exercise as much. I would ride my bike down to the market instead of driving the mile. I would bring back the milk or the loaf of bread on the handlebars. Of course, there was a bit of a problem when I was giving a dinner party and tried to ride back with all the dinner ingredients. Do you have any idea how hard it is to ride a bike while balancing eight bags of groceries on the handlebars?

Sports are also a great way to burn some calories in a fun way. When my kids were younger, they always wanted me to play baseball with them. Using my usual cunning, I devised a way to stay connected with them and not actually have to play or exert any energy. They would be the players, and I would be the spectators. I even went so far as to have a guy dress up like a hot dog vendor and sell me hot dogs while I watched them. The only exercise I really got was during the seventh inning stretch when I would occasionally start a wave.

Getting that Extra Support an Athlete Needs

It's very important to be around people who support your lifestyle and encourage you, even though it's essentially up to you for success. I was amazed that people would know I was trying to take better care of myself, and then offer me cake or just a taste of food that they thought was delicious. They would say, "Don't be ridiculous, a taste is not going to hurt you."

Once again, I'd say, "If I were an alcoholic, would you tell me that one sip of a gin and tonic won't hurt? Or ask me to just have one glass of wine?"

They immediately got my point, and it never happened twice with the same person. People's attitudes about you change when you are thin. Mostly I'm talking about strangers. When you're thin, you're treated as though you're more competent, more intelligent, more talented. I used to play at the Hollywood Stars night in Los Angeles at Dodger Stadium. It was a fun game of baseball played by celebrities before the real Dodgers Game. It was awesome being on the field and looking up and seeing thousands of fans. But when I was fat, I never got to actually play in the game. I was the celebrity bench warmer. The athletic actors, like Tom Selleck, Mark Harmon, Billy Crystal, and Tony Danza, were the players. The one year I played after I lost weight was the only time I actually got up to bat. I struck out, but it was a great feeling being there. All my practice time at the batting cages didn't pay off, but I had the time of my life. And, being struck out by Tom Selleck—what an honor!

Have You Seen a Doctor? No, Just Dots

During my first session at the gym, the instructor asked me, "How many dots do you do?" I thought he was talking about my favorite movie theatre candy. I said, "About 2 boxes, but if it's a double feature I could do more."

Eventually, I learned he was talking about the Stairmaster. When I first started, I thought "My God, I can only do 3 dots in 10 minutes." I learned to hate those dots. Now I just cover them up because I don't want to even know how many dots I have to go. It's kind of like losing weight in general. Start off at your own pace and eventually increase it. I used to look over at the person next to me to see how many dots they were doing, but I've realized it doesn't matter. They're not the one trying to lose my weight—I am. Besides, soon the endorphins kick in and that extra dot is quite a bit closer.

I can't tell you how many times over the years I have thrown in the towel on my latest diet and said to myself, "I'm fat. I'm going to be fat my whole life, and I'm just going to learn to love myself." But I couldn't love myself because I hated myself. I hated being fat. I hated that I knew I was taking years off my life and accepting it.

I'll be at the gym and I'll see someone really obese and I want to go up and hug them. I want to say, "You know what? I think it's so wonderful what you're doing, and it can be done." To me, it's much more impressive to see a woman who weighs 250 pounds on the Stairmaster than it is to see the aerobics queen with the matching headband and the leotards up the butt. (Now a 250-pound woman with a leotard up the butt...that's a different subject.)

Chapter Thirteen

Is It Getting Complicated in Here?

You may have seen a video that I made with the American Diabetes Association called *D4G* (*Diabetes for Guys*). We made it because guys are guys; we don't want to admit that we're sick, and we don't want to take care of ourselves. The video was fun to do because we played around with a lot of my favorite movies—and some of my favorite movie spoofs ended up on the cutting-room floor. But the reason we made it was to get your attention. I wanted to encourage everyone by getting them to laugh at diabetes skits in the guise of *Forrest Gump* or *A Few Good Men*. I wanted to plant some simple ideas for ways you can take better care of yourself while you're living with diabetes.

I found out I had diabetes on a routine college entrance physical. It was no surprise to

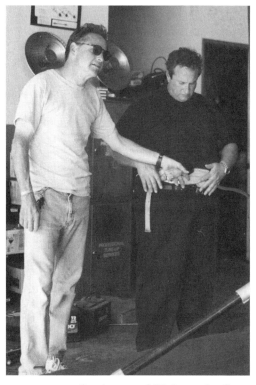

On the set of *Diabetes for Guys*

anyone in the medical profession that I would be a prime candidate for diabetes. I weighed about 300 pounds, and my father had just died of diabetes complications. They were suspicious, so they gave me a glucose tolerance test. They told me to drink this lemony syrup and said that it wouldn't taste that good, but I had to drink the whole thing. I thought it tasted great. As a matter of fact, I asked if they had an extra one.

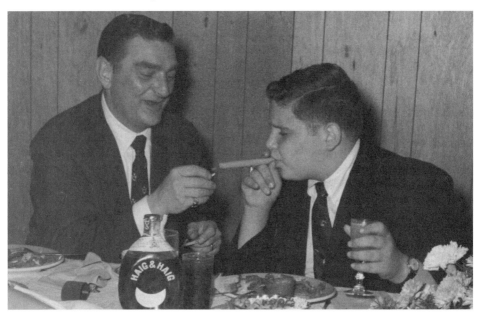

Dad and me at my Bar Mitzvah. (Obviously, two very healthy guys!)

I was devastated when I found out I had diabetes. It scared me to death for about 2 weeks, then I continued my fat life as if I never heard the news. I knew my dad had diabetes. He weighed 260 pounds. He was a funny man and liked to make us laugh, but I don't remember him ever taking care of himself. He'd say, "I'll eat this, and I'll just shoot up another 5 units of insulin." It was kind of a Russian roulette. Sometimes the insulin was just right; sometimes he'd give himself too much insulin. Most of the time he'd start shaking and stuff, just to scare and entertain us. And then once he was really shaking and had to tell us to go get mom!

I wasn't afraid of the needle when I had to take insulin injections, but I was very haphazard about it. I'd sometimes get dressed and realize that I hadn't taken my shot, so I'd shoot right through my shirt. Real haphazard. But if you have to take insulin to control your blood sugar better, let me tell you, the needles are so micro-thin nowadays that you don't even feel it.

When I'm Feeling Low

I never really had low blood sugar when I was overweight. Now that I'm thinner, I have had that unfortunate experience. Sometimes I'll go long periods without eating if I'm directing or acting, and the low blood sugar will kick in. It's especially bad if I go and work out at the gym. My knees will get wobbly, and I'll think, "Whoa, get some food." If I take my oral medication and don't eat and then I exercise, I can guarantee that I'm going to have a low reaction. Don't do what I do.

To treat low blood sugar, I eat! But I'm so attuned to not eating bad things that I won't go for a candy bar. I'll do the orange juice thing, which I've learned is better than the candy bar. Orange juice has natural sugar—which is carbohydrate—and it goes to work raising your blood sugar faster.

The Pressure is Getting to Me

When I was dieting, I never really counted calories. I'd look at the carb content and the fat content. I never paid attention to the sodium, which now I know I should've because I have high blood pressure. Even with weight loss, healthy eating, and daily exercise—which lowers blood pressure—mine is still high. Now I'm on high blood pressure medication and I'm supposed to watch my sodium. That's a bad combination—diabetes and high blood pressure. It can do damage to your kidneys and blood vessels that you don't even want to think about.

Complications Plain and Simple

Diabetic complications scare people. And you can't blame them; they're scary things. No one wants to lose a foot or their vision. No man wants to lose his ability to, ahem, perform. Now people are saying cigarettes can cause impotence, too (that should help people stop smoking—smoking and diabetes are the worst combination). I haven't had all the complications of diabetes, and I've yet to suffer from sexual dysfunction. I've been lucky.

On the other hand, I have had a taste of some other complications. I've got neuropathy in my feet (which is how I came to lose the weight), so I can't run, because of the nerve damage in my left foot. I would like to be able to run. And I've had some eye problems, so I've experienced laser surgery and am glad to say that it works! I've also been spilling a bit of protein in my urine, so I'm taking an ACE inhibitor for that. It's not unusual to spill a little protein after this length of time with diabetes; the filters in your kidneys get tired. But I get them checked once a year and my doctor keeps an eye on it.

Checking Blood Sugar

We didn't have blood glucose meters when I was first diagnosed with diabetes. At that time, we used test tape, which gave results in a very gray area...it was not very accurate. It can only tell you if your blood sugar was high a couple of hours ago.

I want to make myself believe that I'm so aware of what I'm eating and when I exercise that I don't need to test. But sometimes I get surprised. For example, in the hospital—I'd had no movement, I was always in a bed, and I was on a very low-calorie diet. They'd check my sugar, and it'd be 230! "WHAT?" They'd explain to me that I had eaten an apple on the tray. Or I was under a lot of stress lying there, worrying. It sounds funny, but sometimes stress raises blood sugar more than eating carbs!

I have started checking my sugar with this great new meter that has built in test strips. I don't have to mess with taking the strips out of the bottle, etc. I know; it can be a real pain to have to do this stuff sometimes.

If you have type 2 diabetes, a check when you wake up in the morning to see how your diabetes program is going is usually just about all you need. If you're trying a new medication, you might check two hours after the first bite of a meal to see if your blood sugar is coming back down to where it's supposed to be. If you're starting to exercise more, you might check after you exercise. Exercise can lower your blood sugar just like diabetes pills and insulin can. And exercise has a lowering effect for the next 24 hours, too.

If I Only Knew Then...

I know that when I was first diagnosed, I was scared for about two weeks, and then I said, "So what. I'll get a little tired, or I won't eat the second ice cream." If only I could have had the knowledge and experience of complications I have now. If only I was smart enough at 17...which at 17, you know, you think you're invincible. Which is why 17-year-olds race cars and do dangerous things. But I wish I could change things in my life. Yes, I do. I wish I hadn't grown up weighing 300 pounds. My life would be considerably different now, I think. I'm positive for the better. But I really—without being negative—I really do have regrets. I think everybody has regrets about some decisions they've made. And some people say, "Oh, I would do it all over again," but I wouldn't. I'd take better care of myself.

There are a lot of teenagers developing type 2 diabetes in the United States these days. They say it's because we have too much high-fat food and not enough exercise. Well, yes, that's certainly how I met up with diabetes. But in my day, type 2 diabetes was rarely seen in young people. Now, they're calling it an epidemic. The medical experts also say that a huge research study shows that changing your diet and getting more physical activity can PREVENT diabetes. I sure wish I had known that.

I have a good life. I've been very fortunate. Of course, I wish I didn't have neuropathy. Whenever I cut my foot, half the time it gets infected and I end up in the hospital. I don't know if I'm strong enough to live as an amputee. But I also think that people do what they have to do. Because of diabetes, I've slowly developed a limp in my left leg. I didn't even notice it until I saw myself on the screen. I think I was more depressed about that than actually finding out that I had diabetes. But it's an appearance thing that, as an actor, concerns me.

The Eyes Have It

I have to say though, fortune has smiled on me. I've actually had miraculous luck with my eyes. I get yearly dilated eye exams from my ophthalmologist. Any time I have a problem, I have a laser treatment, and then a month later, they're better. I'm good about having them checked. In fact, I'm really good about the checkups for all the complications. I know that finding them early means treatment is much more likely to be successful.

Using Diabetes to Lose Weight?

I did get down to 217 one time, the bad kind of way—by letting my blood sugar run too high. But as soon as I went on insulin, my weight went back up to 260. Was that depressing? Yeah. It's hard to balance food and insulin or diabetes pills, but I have to eat. I figured it out, and lost the weight. And now I don't need the insulin anymore.

I'm not God though. Sometimes I overeat. I ordered one of those cheeseless pizzas, which would be low-fat, right? Yeah, well, I ate the WHOLE thing. I was sick. I had a stomachache. But I was in a hotel room alone, and I was bored to death. Do these excuses sound familiar? So, the next day you start fresh...

Inspiration

My sister told me that she had my picture on her refrigerator; that I was her inspiration. You have no idea how that feels. I am hoping the best for my sister. She has Murphy's Law with diabetes—if you can get a complication, she's got it. She's currently in the hospital, getting ready to start dialysis.

As for myself, I'm frustrated that it took me so long to get my act together. My doctor says that I've probably added 10 years to my life. There was a time when I was so miserable that I didn't want those 10 years. But now, I'm happy to say, I do!

Do I hope for a cure for diabetes and perhaps a reversal of my complications? I hope, but I don't

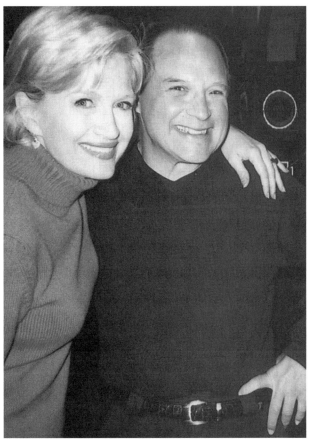

The "New" Stephen with Diane Sawyer

think that'll happen in my lifetime. I do know a person with diabetes who had a pancreas and kidney transplant, and he does not have diabetes any more. I'm wondering why doesn't everybody do this? (I know that the drugs you have to take to suppress your immune system after a transplant can be so toxic, it's a toss-up between which one is harder to live with.) But I did reverse some of my complications by getting better control of the diabetes. Some you can reverse, some you can't. I got some feeling back in my feet, and it hasn't gotten any worse. And the protein that was spilling from my kidneys—that's stopped, too.

The Great American Way

I recently saw a 20/20 episode about how after we get married and live together for awhile, we start to put on weight. It rang true to me. Almost every single one of my friends has gained weight over the years. These are people I used to admire, people whose physiques I envied. Now I am thinnest of all. Oh God, all the teasing that went on, even when I was an adult with other adults. I must say the fact that I am thinner today than they are is the sweetest revenge of all. I don't tease them about their weight because I've been there, but they know, they know...

And so I leave you with a little piece of wisdom that has come to be my motto: "Life is too short. Why make it any shorter by not taking care of yourself?"

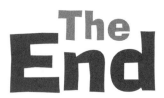

The End

If you liked this **book,** check out **Stephen's video!**

Diabetes for Guys: A Guy Flick

Regular Price: $17.95
Format: VHS
Running Time: 45 minutes
Order number: 4848-01

Please note that this video is for adults, not children.

Stephen and actor Stuart Pankin come together to star in this humorous, sarcastic, slapstick "guy" comedy. Stephen narrates as Stuart mimics his buddy's former life as a 320-pound couch potato who gorges on pizza, beer, and junk food. Simple, hilarious vignettes recreated from films like *Mission Impossible*, *Psycho*, *Austin Powers*, and other popular flicks parody Stephen's evil ways and demonstrate the point of good diabetes management in an exaggerated way. A must-see video!

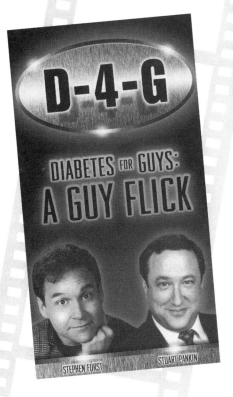

To order by phone, call 1-800-ADA-ORDER and mention the order number, or visit the ADA online store at http://store.diabetes.org (there's no need to use www when typing in this address).

About the American Diabetes Association

The American Diabetes Association is the nation's leading voluntary health organization supporting diabetes research, information, and advocacy. Its mission is to prevent and cure diabetes and to improve the lives of all people affected by diabetes. The American Diabetes Association is the leading publisher of comprehensive diabetes information. Its huge library of practical and authoritative books for people with diabetes covers every aspect of self-care—cooking and nutrition, fitness, weight control, medications, complications, emotional issues, and general self-care.

To order American Diabetes Association books: Call 1-800-232-6733. http://store.diabetes.org [Note: there is no need to use www when typing this particular Web address]

To join the American Diabetes Association: Call 1-800-806-7801. www.diabetes.org/membership

For more information about diabetes or ADA programs and services: Call 1-800-342-2383. E-mail: Customerservice@diabetes.org www.diabetes.org

To locate an ADA/NCQA Recognized Provider of quality diabetes care in your area: www.ncqu.org/dprp/

To find an ADA Recognized Education Program in your area: Call 1-888-232-0822. www.diabetes.org/recognition/education.asp

To join the fight to increase funding for diabetes research, end discrimination, and improve insurance coverage: Call 1-800-342-2383. www.diabetes.org/advocacy

To find out how you can get involved with the programs in your community: Call 1-800-342-2383. See below for program Web addresses.

American Diabetes Month: Educational activities aimed at those diagnosed with diabetes—month of November. www.diabetes.org/ADM

American Diabetes Alert: Annual public awareness campaign to find the undiagnosed—held the fourth Tuesday in March. www.diabetes.org/alert

The Diabetes Assistance & Resources Program (DAR): diabetes awareness program targeted to the Latino community. www.diabetes.org/DAR

African American Program: diabetes awareness program targeted to the African American community. www.diabetes.org/africanamerican

Awakening the Spirit: Pathways to Diabetes Prevention & Control: diabetes awareness program targeted to the Native American community. www.diabetes.org/awakening

To find out about an important research project regarding type 2 diabetes: www.diabetes.org/ada/research.asp

To obtain information on making a planned gift or charitable bequest: Call 1-888-700-7029. www.diabetes.org/ada/plan.asp

To make a donation or memorial contribution: Call 1-800-342-2383. www.diabetes.org/ada/cont.asp